Opioids - From Analgesic Use to Addiction

Edited by Pilar Almela Rojo

Published in London, United Kingdom

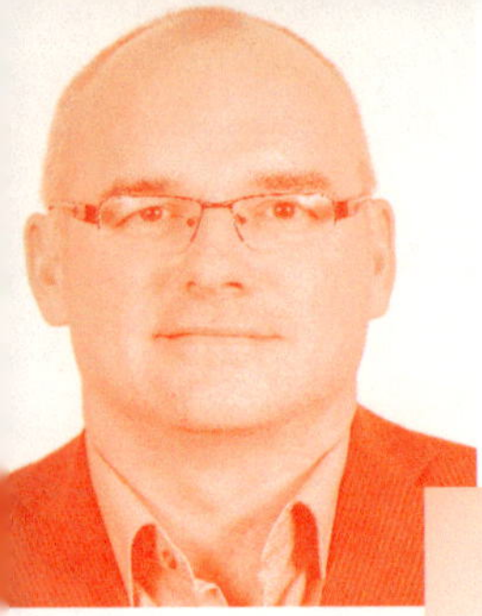
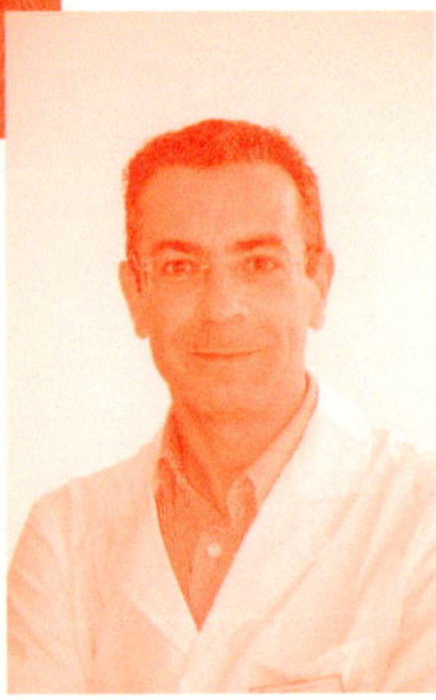
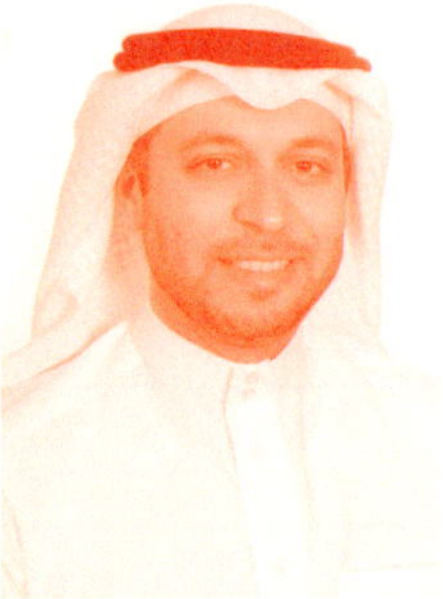
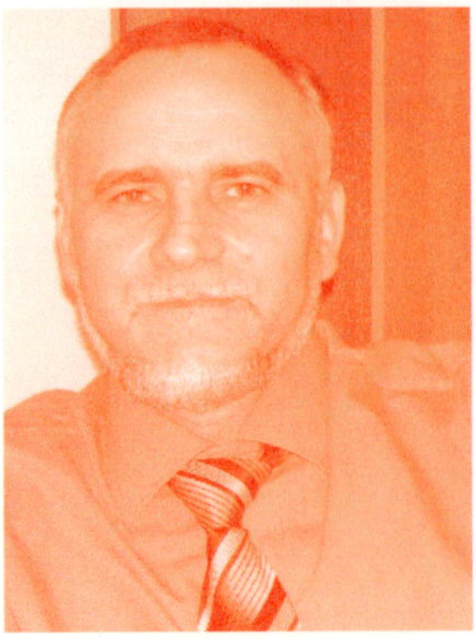
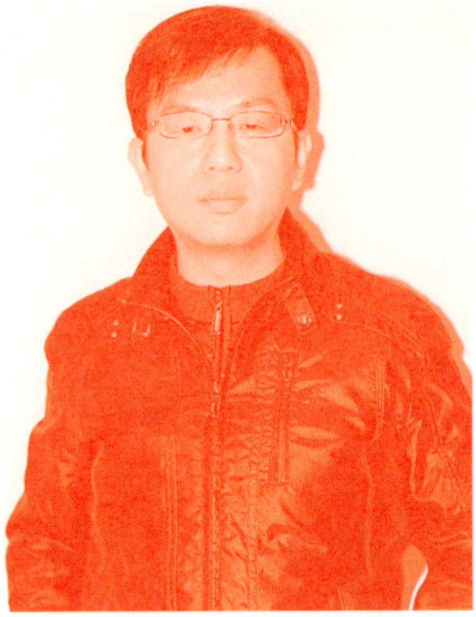
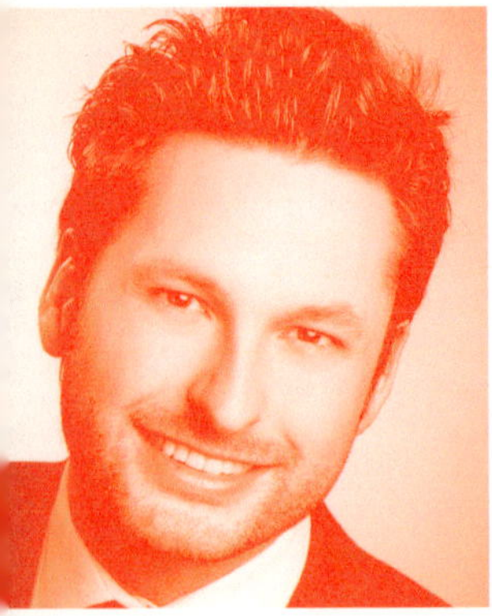
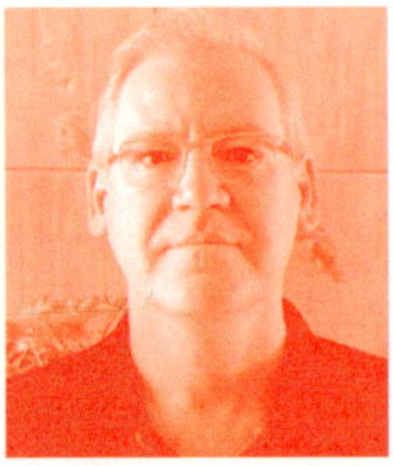

IntechOpen

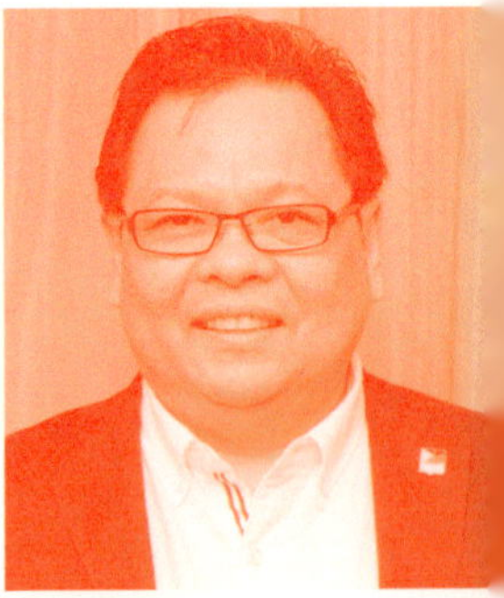
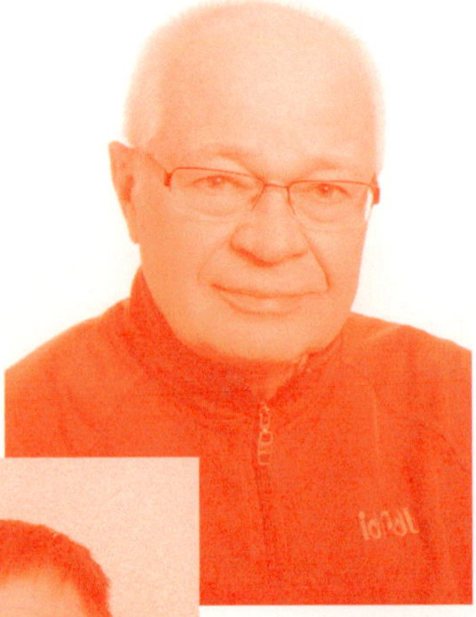
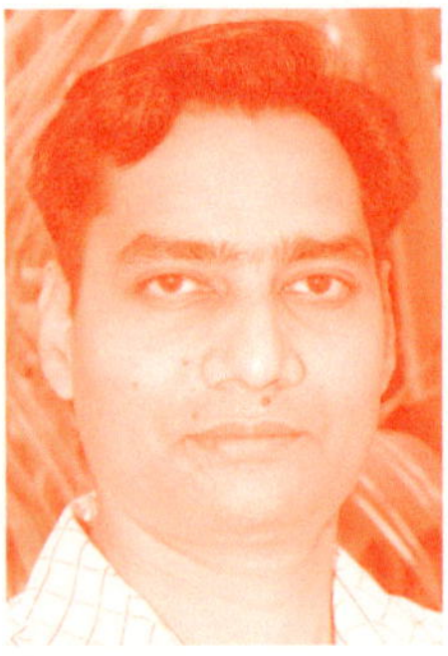
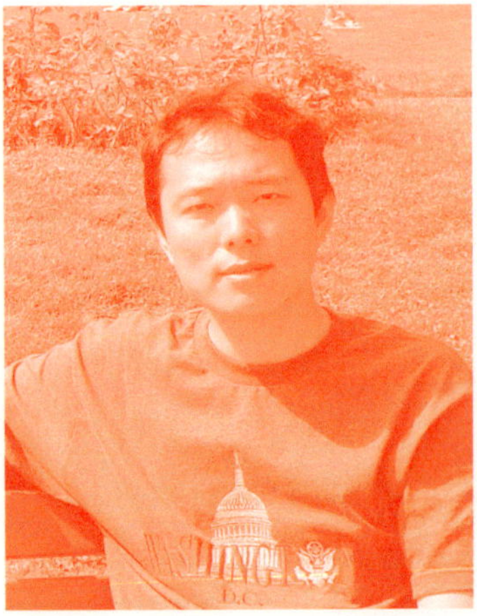
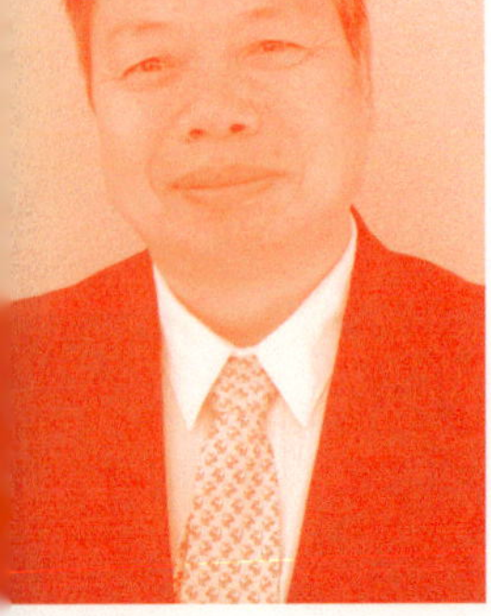
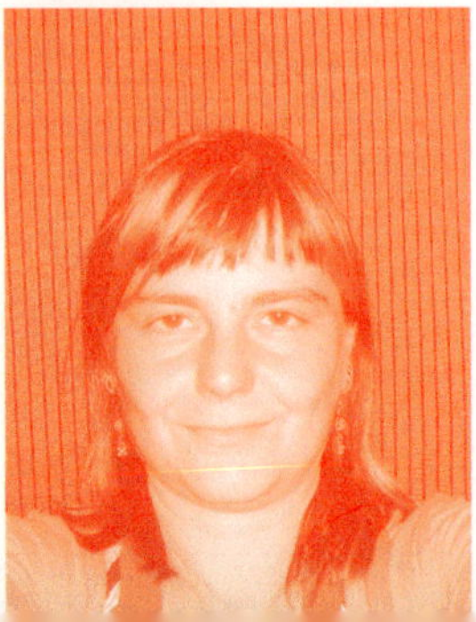

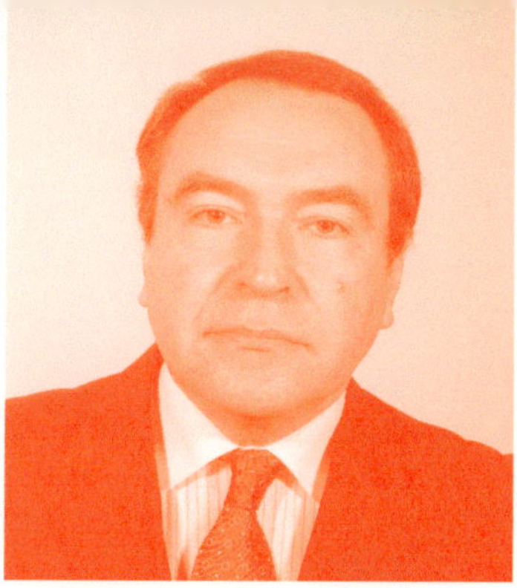
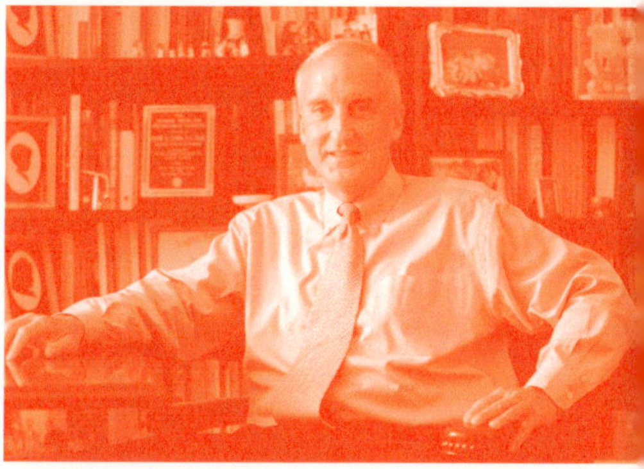
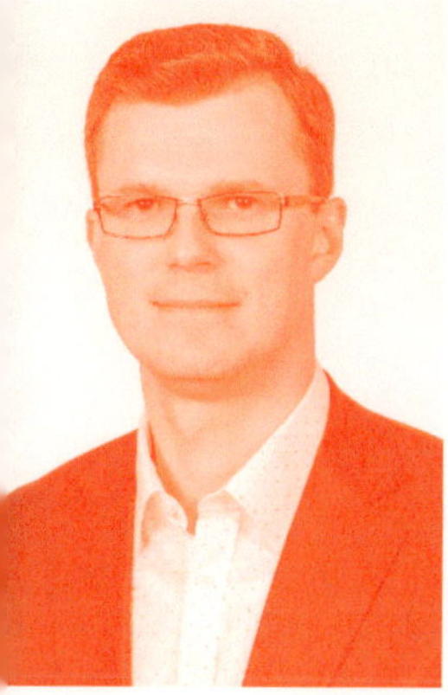
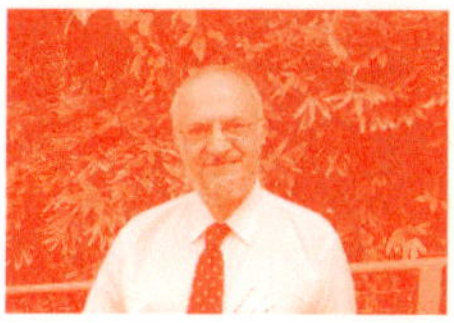
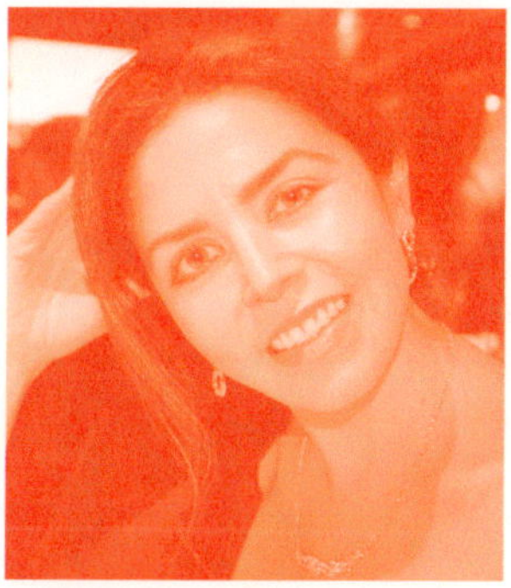

Supporting open minds since 2005

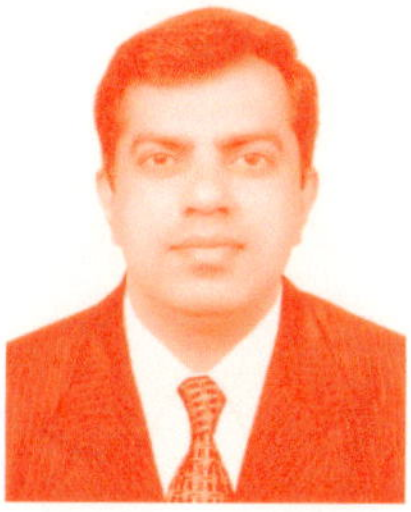
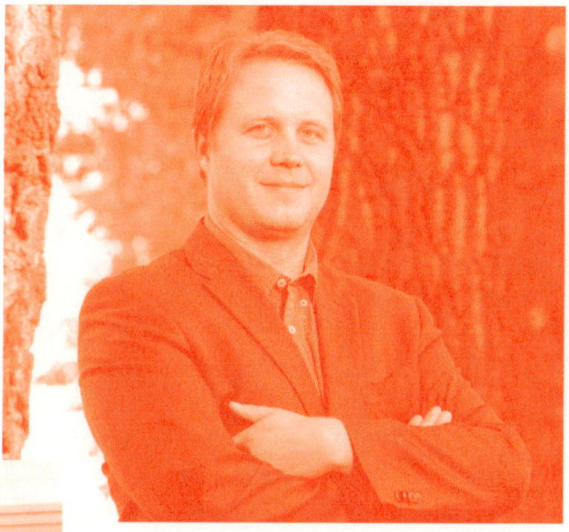
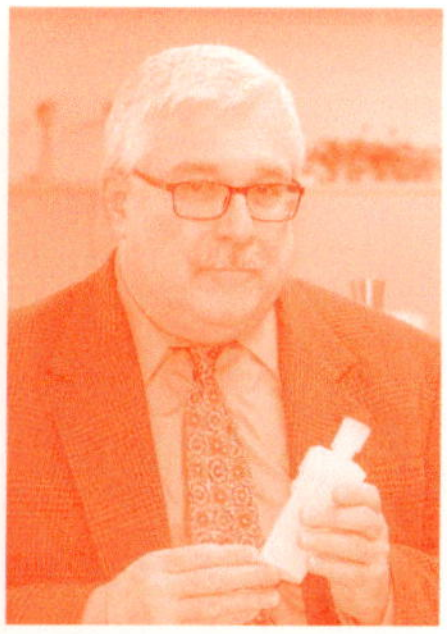
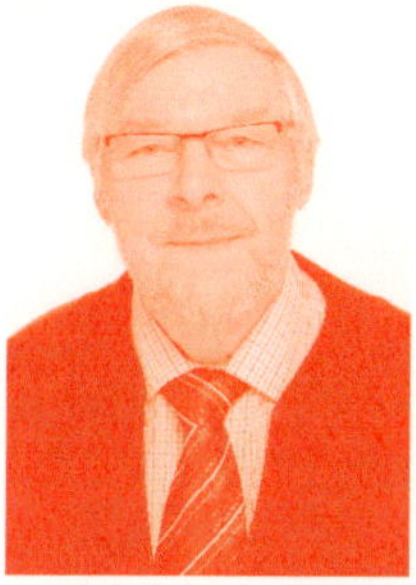
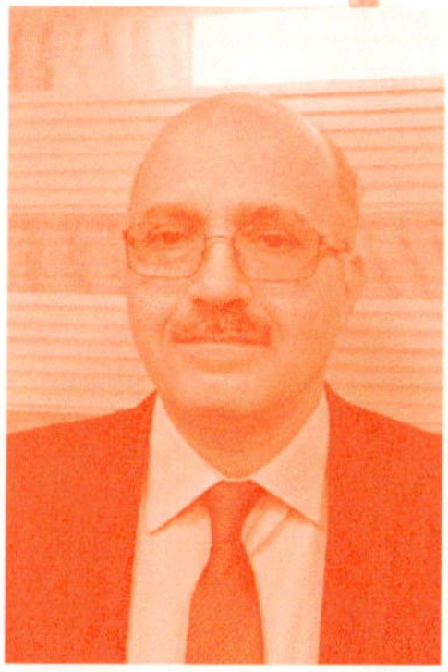
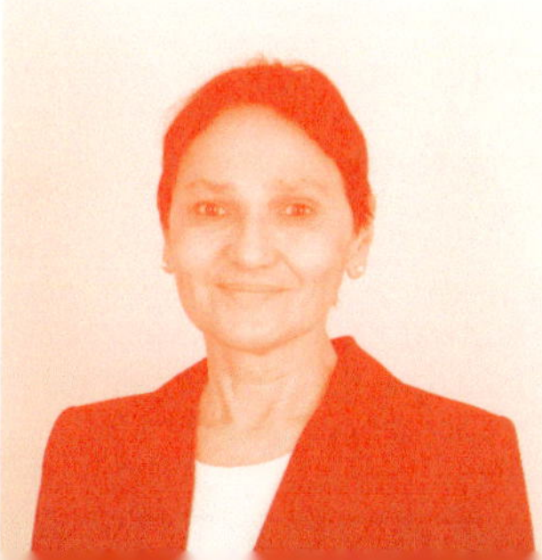
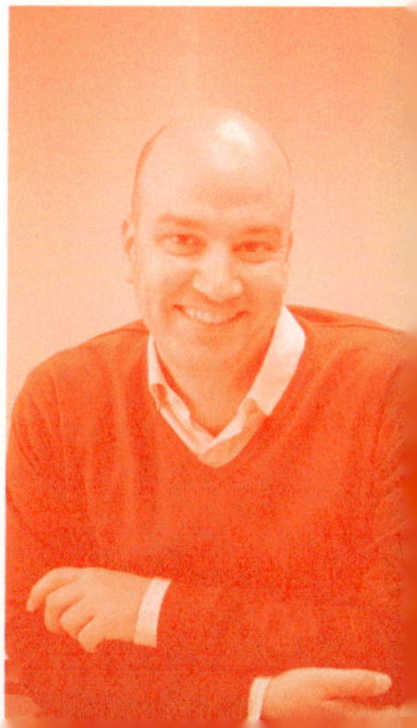

Opioids - From Analgesic Use to Addiction
http://dx.doi.org/10.5772/intechopen.73905
Edited by Pilar Almela Rojo

Contributors
Pilar Almela Rojo, M. Luisa Laorden, Juan Antonio García-Carmona, Elena Martínez-Laorden, María Victoria Milanés, Javier Navarro-Zaragoza, M. Victoria Milanés, Marta Rodriguez-Arias, M Carmen Blanco-Gandia, Sandra Montagud-Romero, Shrenik Ostwal, Pamela Bolyanatz

First published in London, United Kingdom, 2020 by IntechOpen
IntechOpen is the global imprint of INTECHOPEN LIMITED, registered in England and Wales, registration number: 11086078, 7th floor, 10 Lower Thames Street, London, EC3R 6AF, United Kingdom
Printed in Croatia

British Library Cataloguing-in-Publication Data
A catalogue record for this book is available from the British Library

Additional hard and PDF copies can be obtained from orders@intechopen.com

Opioids - From Analgesic Use to Addiction
Edited by Pilar Almela Rojo
p. cm.
Print ISBN 978-1-83880-958-4
Online ISBN 978-1-83880-953-9
eBook (PDF) ISBN 978-1-83880-954-6

For EU product safety concerns:
IN TECH d.o.o., Prolaz Marije Krucifikse Kozulić 3, 51000 Rijeka, Croatia, info@intechopen.com or visit our website at intechopen.com.

Meet the editor

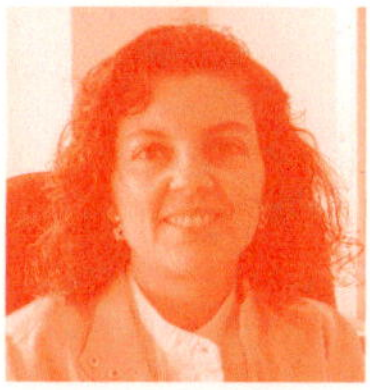

After completing her studies in Pharmacy at the University of Granada, Pilar Almela joined a PhD program in Experimental Biomedical Sciences at the University of Murcia in the Department of Pharmacology, under Professor Laorden's supervision, where she studied different pathway involvement in the adaptive changes observed during morphine dependence. Her training was completed with stays at research centers in USA, France, United Kingdom and Spain. Results from her laboratory have given rise to numerous international publications. These findings can improve the knowledge of mechanisms involved in addiction and establish new prevention and treatment strategies. In 2019, she became an Associate Professor at the Department of Pharmacology, focusing her current research on the design of new nanoparticulate systems for morphine administration.

Contents

Preface

Over the past two decades, some countries have observed an increase in the use of opioid drugs for pain management, including non-oncological pain. The use of prescription opioids is sometimes justified to decrease or abolish the nociceptive sensation but the misuse of this kind of drug, the rise in heroin consumption, and the escalation in the abuse of high-potency synthetic opioids, such as fentanyl, have led to the declaration of an opioid epidemic.

Nowadays, morphine and other opioid drugs are widely used for pain relief in many conditions but their use is associated with potential complications. For example, opioids can produce a rebound effect and cause more pain instead of relief and they have a high chance of generating tolerance, dependence, and addiction, a brain disease induced by repeated or chronic use of these drugs that causes adaptive or allostatic changes (i.e. cellular or system adaptations) that modify the neuronal circuitry, inducing a "drug-dependent" state. This state persists even after drug consumption and affects the feeling of well-being, learning, stress, decision-making, and self-control.

This book is written by international scientists with expertise in psychobiology, addiction, and pain management, and addresses different aspects of opioids, such as understanding central pain and central sensitization for better patient care, effectiveness of morphine in other conditions apart from pain control, neurobiological mechanisms associated with opioid addiction, and pharmacological treatments for this disease.

With this book culminates an intense project in which I would first like to highlight the involvement of all authors who have contributed to a text of great quality and scientific rigor. I would like to thank Ms Romina Rovan, Ms Rozmari Marijan and Ms Manuela Gabric, the Author Service Managers for this book at IntechOpen, for their assistance during book preparation. Finally, I would also like to dedicate this book to my mentor, Professor María Luisa Laorden, and to my family, without any of them, it would not have been possible to get here.

Pilar Almela Rojo
Associate Professor,
Department of Pharmacology,
Faculty of Medicine,
University of Murcia,
Spain

Section 1

General Considerations

Chapter 1

Introductory Chapter: Opioid Analgesics - History, Uses and Risks

Pilar Almela

1. Introduction

Opiates have been used for various purposes throughout history [1, 2] (**Figure 1**). Interest in opium poppy plant (*Papaver somniferum*) arose more than 4500 years ago, due to the nutritional power of its seeds. Afterwards, around 1550 BC, opium was used in the Eastern Mediterranean and Egypt for religious and medicinal purposes. Greek medicine was the first to refer to opium as a narcotic, and it is at this time that a classification of the various preparations of this plant begins. In the seventeenth century, its use as a pain reliever in Sydenham's laudanum began to become general, until it was replaced by the currently used morphine hydrochloride.

In 1803, the German pharmacist, Friedrich Wilhelm Adam Sertürner, identified and isolated the major psychoactive agent in opium, at approximately 4–21% and named it "morphium," alluding to the Greek god of dreams Morpheus [3]. Sertürner and three young assistant experimented the narcotic effects of morphine by taking the raw material. From this moment on, morphine began to be used for the same cases in which opium was used through different routes of administration (oral, rectal, or transdermal). Twenty years after Sertürner's discovery, in 1820, a pharmacist named Heinrich Emmanuel Merck began to commercialize morphine. The medical use of morphine was widespread after the discovery of the hypodermic syringe in the mid-nineteenth century.

In 1973, three independent research groups headed by Solomon Snyder in Baltimore, Eric Simon in New York, and Lars Terenius in Sweden confirmed the existence of specific opioid receptors [4–6], and, 2 years later, Hughes discovered the presence of endogenous peptides able of activating the same receptors, although in a less intense way [7].

The endogenous opioid system plays a main role in multiple physiological functions of the organism. When people carry out certain daily activities (eating, exercising, sexual behavior and others), endogenous opioids are released, inducing a brain reward effect that increases the likelihood that these behaviors tend to repeat. It is the so-called behavioral reinforcing effect, which can lead to addictive behaviors.

Nowadays, morphine is widely used for chronic to severe pain relief in many conditions associated with heart attacks, serious injury, postoperative discomfort, and terminal illness such as cancer [8]. However, it is not possible to uncouple its beneficial analgesic effect from addiction, tolerance, and dependence. Being able to separate the potent analgesia from the addictive capacity would make pain relief to be a minor medical problem.

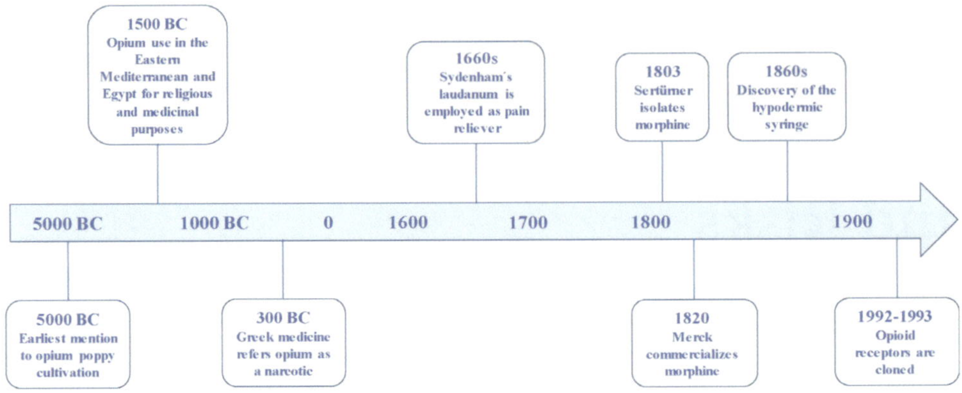

Figure 1.
Timeline of morphine history.

2. Opioid receptors

There are three main opioid receptor types that produce pharmacologic effects upon stimulation, mu (MOP), kappa (KOP), and delta (DOR), and morphine is a MOR-preferring agonist. The novel nociception/orphanin FQ receptor is considered to be a non-opioid branch of the opioid receptor family (**Figure 2**). However, substantial pharmacological evidence for additional opioid receptor phenotypes exists [9].

Opioid receptors are a group of G_i/G_o protein-coupled receptors, which consist of seven transmembrane domains, three extracellular, and three intracellular loops, extracellular amino acid N-terminus, and intracellular carboxyl C-terminus. They are activated both by endogenously opioid peptides and by exogenously administered natural, synthetic, or semisynthetic opiate compounds such as morphine and heroin.

Opioid receptors are located in both the central and peripheral nervous system. Morphine analgesia is mainly due to its action on MOP receptors, although the activation of KOP and DOP receptors also participates in the analgesic effects of this drug. These receptors act synergistically in different places at CNS level, from the spinal cord to the cerebral cortex, inhibiting the nociceptive sensation whatever its location or intensity. Specifically, they act on the afferent system at the spinal level, where the activation of MOP receptors results in the inhibition of primary sensory fibers. Morphine also acts by regulating the transmission of the efferent system, inhibiting the nociceptive transmission sent from mesencephalic areas and the brainstem. Nevertheless, opiates not only diminish the painful sensation but also

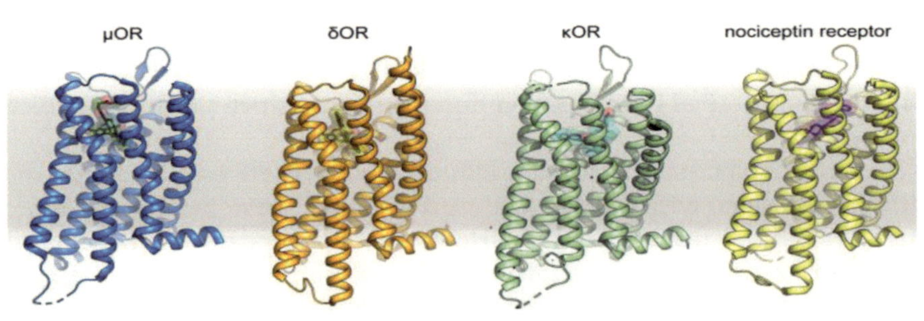

Figure 2.
Opioid receptor structures. Modified from [10].

block the unpleasant or distressing feelings that accompany pain through its action at the limbic and cortical level, areas involved in emotional physiological responses and where a large number of opioid receptors are expressed.

Some pharmacological properties of opioid agonists are routinely used in clinic practice. In addition to the aforementioned opioid analgesic power, these drugs have utility in other conditions as cough suppressant, antidiarrheal, emetic, and anesthetics, being also used in special situations as in the acute pulmonary edema or in respiratory rhythm regulation in patients undergoing artificial respiration.

3. Genetic polymorphisms modulating the pain response

Recent research in the field of pharmacogenomics has discovered important single-nucleotide polymorphisms that are thought to be linked to opioid dose variability. This could explain the genetic changes in the analgesic opioid dose. These polymorphisms appear in several areas involved in pain pathways, drug receptors, drug-metabolizing enzymes, and drug efflux molecules [11]. Among the genetic polymorphisms identified as possible modulators of the pain response, we can mention genes that code for voltage-gated sodium channels, the metabolic enzyme catechol-O-methyltransferase (COMT), the synthetic enzyme CTP cyclohydrolase, and the changes described in the OPRM1 gene [12].

A better knowledge of these polymorphisms can help clinicians to manage interindividual variability in opioid demands. These genetic markers could also help to design tools to precisely predict the analgesic opioid dose, increase efficacy, and reduce the incidence of drug dependence and addiction.

4. Opioid addiction: a severe substance use disorder

Today, morphine is a Schedule II narcotic, along with other drugs like fentanyl, hydromorphone, meperidine, methadone, or oxycodone, under the Controlled Substances Act (US Drug Enforcement Administration) [13], and is available only by a prescription due to its high potential for abuse. Morphine is also regulated because it is the precursor to heroin, a synthetic alkaloid that presents a different pharmacokinetics than morphine, resulting in more acute CNS effects, partly responsible for the tremendous addictive capacity of this molecule.

The first experiences with opioids are usually unpleasant, since the effects on the gastrointestinal tract (nausea and vomiting) predominate. However, when repeating the behavior, tolerance to the emetic action develops, then the feeling of euphoria prevails.

The addictive state is characterized by the compulsive consumption of the drug despite the serious negative consequences that it entails, such as diseases, neglecting social and family obligations, and the need to commit criminal acts to obtain the substance. For drug addicts, drugs become the main incentive within their scale of values, and, as a result, their lives are reduced to obtaining and consuming drugs.

In addition, drug addiction involves loss of control in limiting intake and emerging of a negative emotional state (e.g., dysphoria, anxiety and irritability), reflecting a motivational withdrawal syndrome when access to the drug is prevented [14].

The addictive process consists of three stages (**Figure 3**): binge/intoxication, withdrawal/negative affect, and preoccupation/anticipation (craving). These stages interact with each other, becoming more intense and ultimately leading to the state known as addiction.

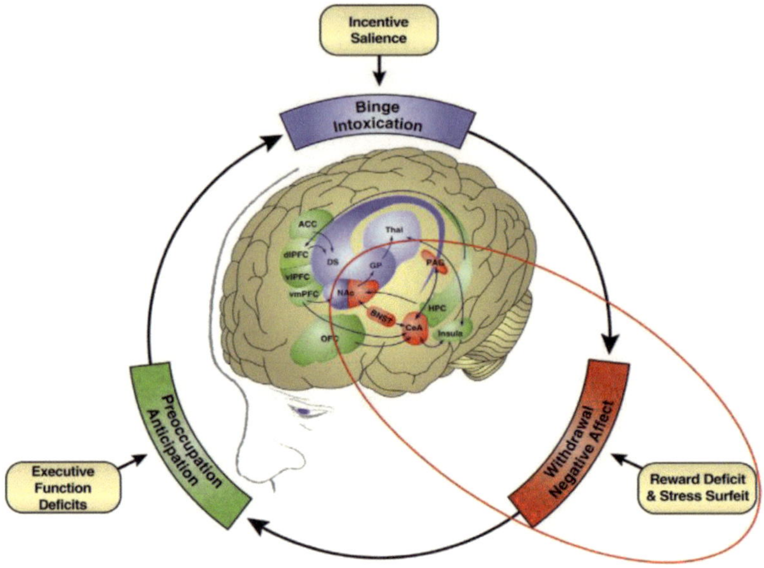

Figure 3.
Neurobiological bases of substance use disorders [14].

In the Diagnostic and Statistical Manual of Mental Disorders (DSM-5), addiction is synonymous with a severe substance use disorder, and opioid use disorder is included here [15]. Just like it happens with other substance use disorders, individuals can begin opioid misuse with recreational use of the drug and evolve to the withdrawal/negative affect stage as negative reinforcement appear.

Despite numerous treatment attempts and the serious risk to their lives, relapses to drug-seeking and drug-taking behaviors following months or years of abstinence are frequent when addicts find stimuli associated with the first contact with the drug [16]. This fact shows that we need more effective long-term treatments for drug dependence and emphasizes, on the other hand, the importance of better understanding the neurobiological mechanisms that underlie drug addiction and their persistence.

5. The opioid epidemic: challenges and opportunities

Over the past 20 years, there has been a significant increase in opioid prescription worldwide, but especially in the United States. This substantial increase in opioid prescribing patterns has been due, in part, to the influence of certain currents of opinion, which trivialized the potential drawbacks of opioid painkillers, along with the widely spread belief that any kind of pain could and should be treated with opioids. On the other hand, consuming higher doses than prescribed or by people who had not been prescribed, or switching to a more direct route of administration than the oral route, has contributed to the expansion of the abuse of these drugs among the population [17].

An opioid epidemic has been declared in 2017 in the United States [1, 18]. Europe and, particularly, low- and middle-income countries, appear to be less influenced by this problem. An estimated 10.3 million Americans aged 12 and older misused opioids in 2018, including 9.9 million prescription pain reliever (morphine, oxycodone, and hydrocodone) abusers and 808,000 heroin users. A report from the Centers for Disease Control and Prevention (CDC) indicated that opioid sales multiplied by 14 from 1999 to 2010. Moreover, this center reported that, in 2017, the number of overdose deaths involving opioids (including prescription and illegal opioids) was six times higher than in 1999. Prescription opioid overdose, abuse, and dependence involve high economic costs for American society from around $78.5 billion.

Avoiding prescription of opioid pain relievers when its therapeutic indication is doubtful or unnecessary is always easier than proceeding later upon treatments for abuse, which will be even more difficult if the patient is not involved. Only in certain situations, opioid administration for pain relieve is essential; for all the others, a great diversity of interventions that can be as effective or more than the prescription of opioids are available, avoiding thus the potential risks of addiction and overdose that are associated with the consumption of opiates.

Different states have begun implementing prescription drug monitoring programs to control irregular prescribing practices by clinicians and the recreational use of opioids. In addition, current strategies include a greater involvement of healthcare professionals (such as psychiatrists) and approaches to address comorbidities [19]. These measures could be resulting in a decrease in opioid prescription, as shown in last reports from CDC, which indicate a reduction in these prescriptions from 2016 [20].

Author details

Pilar Almela
Department of Pharmacology, Faculty of Medicine, University of Murcia, Murcia, Spain

*Address all correspondence to: palmela@um.es

References

[1] Devereaux AL, Mercer SL, Cunningham CW. DARK classics in chemical neuroscience: Morphine. ACS Chemical Neuroscience. 2018;**9**:2395-2407. DOI: 10.1021/acschemneuro.8b00150

[2] Presley CC, Lindsley CW. DARK Classics in chemical neuroscience: Opium, a historical perspective. ACS Chemical Neuroscience. 2018;**9**:2503-2518. DOI: 10.1021/acschemneuro.8b00459

[3] Sertürner F. Säure im Opium. Journal Der Pharmacie. 1805;**13**:229-243

[4] Pert CB, Snyder SH. Opiate receptor: Demonstration in nervous tissue. Science. 1973;**179**:1011-1074. DOI: 10.1126/science.179.4077.1011

[5] Simon EJ, Hiller JM, Edelman I. Stereospecific binding of the potent narcotic analgesic [3H]etorphine to rat brain homogenate. Proceedings of the National Academy of Sciences of the United States of America. 1973;**70**:1947-1949. DOI: 10.1073/pnas.70.7.1947

[6] Terenius L. Stereospecific interaction between narcotic analgesics and synaptic plasma membrane fraction of rat cerebral cortex. Acta Pharmacologica et Toxicologica. 1973;**32**:317-320. DOI: 10.1111/j.1600-0773.1973.tb01477.x

[7] Hughes J, Smith TW, Kosterlitz HW, Fothergill LA, Morgan BA, Morrisa HR. Identification of two related pentapeptides from the brain with potent opiate agonist activity. Nature. 1975;**258**:577-579. DOI: 10.1038/258577a0

[8] Sverrisdottir E, Lund TM, Olesen AE, Drewes AM, Christrup LL, Kreilgaard M. A review of morphine and morphine-6-glucuronide's pharmacokinetic-pharmacodynamic relationships in experimental and clinical pain. European Journal of Pharmaceutical Sciences. 2015;**74**:45-62. DOI: 10.1016/j.ejps. 2015.03.020

[9] Waldhoer M, Bartlett SE, Whistler JL. Opioid receptors. Annual Review of Biochemistry. 2004;**73**:953-990. DOI: 10.1146/annurev.biochem.73.011303.073940

[10] Manglik A. Molecular basis of opioid action: From structures to new leads. Biological Psychiatry. 2020;**87**:6-14. DOI: 10.1016/j.biopsych.2019.08.028

[11] Kumar S, Kundra P, Ramsamy K, Surendiran A. Pharmacogenetics of opioids: A narrative review. Anaesthesia. 2019;**74**:1456-1470. DOI: 10.1111/anae.14813

[12] Cornett EM, MAC T, Pinner A, Thakur P, TSG S, Siddaiah H, et al. Pharmacogenomics of pain management: The impact of specific biological polymorphisms on drugs and metabolism. Current Oncology Reports. 2020;**22**:18. DOI: 10.1007/s11912-020-0865-4

[13] U.S. Department of Justice. Drug Enforcement Administration. A DEA Resource Guide. 2017 ed. 2017. Available from: https://www.dea.gov/sites/default/files/sites/getsmartaboutdrugs.com/files/publications/DoA_2017Ed_Updated_6.16.17.pdf#page=45

[14] Koob GF. Neurobiology of opioid addiction: Opponent process, hyperkatifeia, and negative reinforcement. Biological Psychiatry. 2020;**87**:44-53. DOI: 10.1016/j.biopsych.2019.05.023

[15] American Psychiatric Association. Diagnostic and Statistical Manual of Mental Disorders. 5th ed. Washington, DC: American Psychiatric Publishing; 2013

[16] Koob GF, Volkow ND. Neurocircuitry of addiction. Neuropsychopharmacology. 2010;**35**:217-238. DOI: 10.1038/npp.2009.110

[17] Kaye AD, Jones MR, Kaye AM, Ripoll JG, Galan V, Beakley BD, et al. Prescription opioid abuse in chronic pain: An updated review of opioid abuse predictors and strategies to curb opioid abuse: Part 1. Pain Physician. 2017;**20**:S93-S109

[18] Morrow JB, Ropero-Miller JD, Catlin ML, Winokur AD, Cadwallader AB, Staymates JL, et al. The opioid epidemic: Moving toward an integrated, holistic analytical response. Journal of Analytical Toxicology. 2019;**43**:1-9. DOI: 10.1093/jat/bky049

[19] Volkow ND, Blanco C. The changing opioid crisis: Development, challenges and opportunities. Molecular Psychiatry. 2020. DOI: 10.1038/s41380-020-0661-4

[20] Annual Surveillance Report of Drug-Related Risks and Outcomes. United States: CDC National Center for Injury Prevention and Control. 2019. Available from: https://www.cdc.gov/drugoverdose/pdf/pubs/2019-cdc-drug-surveillance-report.pdf

Section 2

Opioid Uses

Chapter 2

A New Paradigm: Prevention of Central Sensitization in Pain Management through Minimizing Opioid Exposure

Pamela Bolyanatz

Abstract

Current exacerbations of chronic pain cannot be understood in isolation from how past incidents impact pain and its experience. Patients who frequent the Emergency Room or hospital for a pain crisis or intensification of their pain without new findings on X-rays or scans are often seen as 'drug seekers.' Yet, to the patient the pain is agonizing, and the suffering real. It is this type of patient that prompted an ongoing improvement project in our local hospital, our Multiple Visit Patient Complex Care Program. The goal was to determine the similarities between this type of 'complex' patient—who frequents the hospital despite no new radiographic change—and other patients. Understanding this 'complex' pattern in terms of central intractable pain can change the trajectory of treatment. Results of our program described here reveal that a better understanding of central pain and central sensitization can result in better patient care.

Keywords: opioids, central sensitization, central intractable pain, trauma, multi-modal pain management

1. Introduction: the costs of misdiagnosing pain

Patient complaints of pain can befuddle even the most experienced healthcare provider. The seeming lack of an organic origin, along with multiple exacerbating affective and cognitive variables can result in stopgap measures and incomplete or inaccurate diagnoses. The costs of this approach to treatment can be significant.

Broadly speaking, misdiagnoses or inadequate contribute to overall runaway healthcare costs. The cost of pain care is exorbitant already; inaccurate diagnoses can result in money spent for the wrong treatment: 'The annual cost of pain was greater than the annual costs in 2010 dollars of heart disease ($309 billion), cancer ($243 billion), and diabetes ($188 billion) and nearly 30% higher than the combined cost of cancer and diabetes' [1].

For individual patients who do not receive an accurate diagnosis of their pain, there is a risk of a redundancy of testing that can result in increased exposure to radiation, risk of further misdiagnosis, and mistreatment. The primary risk to the patient, however, is the development of debility, immobility, and isolation.

The reasons for inadequate pain diagnoses are sometimes attributed to the patients themselves. Many times, patients are labeled as 'drug seekers' when they come to the Emergency Department complaining of pain. If patients are presumed to be drug seekers, and if opiates are the easy default treatment for pain, this combination can easily lead to a resistance, even if not entirely conscious—on the part of healthcare staff to assume that the pain is overstated, or perhaps even utterly absent. The ready use of opiates, then, does have to be seen as a contributing problem to pain misdiagnoses. This predisposition has its own set of costs.

For example, patients may have neurobiological anomalies, in which there is an anxiety, fear, and pain matrix in the prefrontal cortex and amygdala. This is influenced by neurotransmitters and glial cell activation, which can lead to pervasive inflammation and central sensitivity. It is paramount that hospitals utilize non-opioid and multi-modal treatments after surgeries to reduce opioid exposure of the brain. The exposure of the insula and the limbic area of the brain to morphine or hydromorphone begins the cascade of blocking endogenous opioid production.

In fact, ~20% of patients complaining of pain have likely used illicit substances, and may be found to have psychiatric or opioid use disorders that are not accurately diagnosed and miss proper treatment with medical-assisted drug therapy. Sporadic follow-up, and missed opportunities to begin treatment due to the health care providers judgment and stigma, can lead to becoming stuck in the same cycle [2].

Ultimately, it is vital to determine a patient's full history. Displays of judgment that evoke a patient's sense of being stigmatized will more likely lead to an improper diagnosis and treatment by the healthcare team. If a treatment is not effective, then understanding the options to reassess and change the course of treatment become necessary. Opioid administration guidelines have been slowly changing since 2005 with the concept of 'not every increase in pain should be met with a higher dose of narcotics (opioids)' [3]. Further research into hormonal, dietary, and other natural or integrative methods of the treatment of pain is increasingly necessary, especially as the costs of opioid use for misdiagnosed pain become more widely known.

2. Current practices in pain treatment

Today healthcare providers are working to lower opioid use in their own way, some in systemized fashion, while other just draw a line in their practice and hope that patients' pain improves, and/or that the patients get tired of asking for medication. But the use of opioids, especially, in pain management today is a complex landscape.

Pain and the treatment or management of pain is a widely debated subject. It is typically not a favorite topic of most providers; many feel they were not trained to care for the wide variety of pain complaints and some throw their hands up in frustration at the myriad of complaints they hear. Some providers have changed their office policy to include a blanket statement, "I do not prescribe narcotics." The reason for this policy, gleaned through many conversations with providers, is that they prefer to avoid the many 'headaches' from the 'drug seekers.' Case Study 1 illustrates this problem.

Case Study 1

A patient arrives at the Emergency Department with no external presenting problems, but she describes her internal pain as, 'I feel like I am going to break apart.' She had undergone surgery 1 week prior, a straightforward laparoscopic cholecystectomy, but she is sure there is an infection or something worse inside. The staff in the Emergency Room see her often for her anxiety; they have other patients with 'true' emergencies in the rooms next door. Should she receive opioids for her pain? She and others like her struggle with feelings of anxiety, fear, pain and often come to the Emergency Department for relief. On a daily basis, patients with chronic pain feel their pain in a way that is difficult to express to others. Their previous experiences of anxiety, trauma, chronic disease, and previous treatment with opioids influence their current situation.

But medical providers are not the only piece of the puzzle. National pharmacy chains have placed restrictions of 7 days for the first prescription of opioids, regardless of whether the patient is opioid naïve or opioid tolerant. This can have unintended outcomes, exemplified by Case Study 2:

Case Study 2

A postoperative patient changed pharmacies shortly after surgery. He was able to receive the first 7 days of medication, but while the pharmacy was waiting for a phone call to complete his authorization, he did not have access to his regularly prescribed medication. This contributed to a pain crisis and he was hospitalized for 3 days. With his regular opioid medication dosage, the admission could have been prevented. The patient was not misusing his medication; he was affected by a ruling that was put in place to safeguard opioid medication from getting in to the hands of those who do not need a large quantity of opioid medication (from Ref. [3]).

Many state surgical organizations are taking notice of the overprescribing on the part of their members in the past. A not uncommon unintended consequence of this practice has been for post-operative patients, historically, to take a few oral pain relievers, and then the rest of the bottle of hydrocodone (Norco™, Vicodin) or oxycodone (Percocet™) sits in the medicine cupboard for many years. The result is that many household opioid supplies allow patients to self- and over-medicate in ways that "fly under the radar" of healthcare personnel. Case Study 3 is one such instance:

Case Study 3

A patient arrived at the Emergency Room in clear distress from her new onset pneumonia. She was experiencing significant chest discomfort, and asked for pain medications since her hydrocodone with acetaminophen 7.5/325 mg was not working; the patient felt that something stronger was needed, and so insisted on a stronger dose. Emergency Room providers do not routinely administer opioids for pneumonia, so she left the hospital against medical advice, frustrated that her pain was not controlled. She eventually returned due to her worsening pneumonia symptoms, which resulted in hospitalization.

3. Factors that affect the experience of pain

Ossipov et al. [4] found the experience of pain to be influenced by emotions and experiences. Painful experiences accompanied by intense emotions, such as wartime injuries, or co-occurring mental health disorders play a role in the body's own endogenous inhibitory system in heightening the pain perception.

Pain perception and modulation are important concepts to understand within pain management and its treatment, as in **Figure 1**.

The following is not an exhaustive list of some of the complexities of the experience of pain; they are offered to show that today's pain management provider must be something of a jack-of-all-trades in order to understand the nature and treatment of pain.

- *Multiple medications are often utilized in the management of pain*. Antidepressants, anti-inflammatories, and bowel medications are all important parts of the picture. Some are finding that topical treatments can be effective in the treatment of pain. It can be a burden to maintain a working knowledge of the plethora of available options, in order to be able to utilize the most effective pain medications, especially if one is not a pain specialist.

- *There are not enough pain specialists*. There is a disparity between the number of pain specialists and the number of patients in pain. Pain patients sense, not

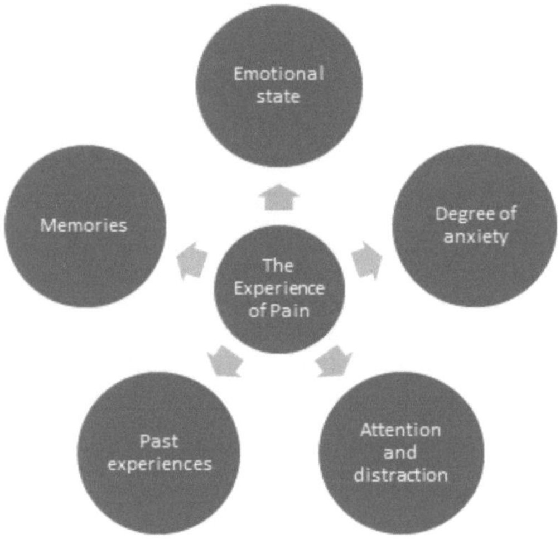

Figure 1.
Factors influencing the pain experience [4].

surprisingly, that their needs are viewed as of secondary importance when they perceive that their sense of urgency is not matched by healthcare team.

- *Patient pain care guidelines do not have individual complex patients in mind.* It is a constant challenge to maintain a targeted therapy for a patient and stay within the morphine milligrams guidelines as set by national and state guidelines. Some states have even prepared guidelines for Emergency Rooms that generalize treatments rather than allow for individual treatments of pain [5].

- *Patient frustration can be high*. Maintaining the provider-patient relationship can be difficult if the non-opioid medications do not work, and the only thing that helps is the opioid pain relievers [6]. The real struggle comes when the opioids are ineffective or requests for more and more opioids occur, especially if a provider is not aware of other options for pain control or even the true diagnosis of the patient. This is exacerbated by the fact that if opioids are overused, the diagnostic picture can become clouded due to suspicion.

- *Patient expectations are based on past history*. Often, when a patient comes to the Emergency Room and has a history of being on chronic opioids, the opioids become the focus of the visit. The struggle begins: the patient feels they deserve more, since their home medications (including, sometimes, that leftover hydrocodone or oxycodone) do not work. For her part, the provider does not want to give opioids, given the growing awareness of opioid-related problems, especially now that providers receive scorecards with their opioid prescribing measured.

- *Surgical delay can limit choices for the orthopedic patient*. Current guidelines for knee replacement are to 'proceed with total joint replacement after **all** other modalities have failed' [7]. This delay may increase the use of opioids since many patients struggle with limited mobility, and perhaps severe pain for many months or years, until they have qualified for the replacement. Ironically, a predisposition to leap to opioids is often done in order to delay the surgery. Recovery is often delayed due to the muscle atrophy of older patients, and these patients often need higher doses of medications to be able to tolerate movement.

- *An increasingly obese population has implications for pain management*. Obesity becomes a post-operative barrier to surgery due to lack of mobility. Physical therapy pain can be more intense and last longer if movement has been difficult for a patient.

The list of considerations entailed in understanding the nature of pain and subsequent pain management could go on. Patients with debilitating illnesses who have had to retire early may be less mobile and so more susceptible to pain—post-operative or other. Clinical observations reveal that back pain and spinal stenosis can leave a patient with weak proximal thigh muscles and the inability to walk more than 30–40 feet, while daily headaches can lead to the inability to leave the home for weeks at a time. Prolonged chronic pain and discomfort often leads to disability.

Disability from pain is increasing. Clinically, patients become more and more deconditioned. They often ambulate or walk less, lose muscle mass, and may become discouraged and often depressed. Some eat lower-quality food, as in the case of a 50-year-old patient who told me that she orders from a mobile app at home and has her food delivered to her, since she cannot drive or stand to cook. Her diet is fast food almost exclusively. This leads to isolation and emotional 'sadness' as described by many patients. Many of the pain patients in my practice state, 'I want to be a good parent (or son, daughter, wife, husband), but I hurt too much.' The psychological and cognitive dysfunction persist.

4. The missing link: central intractable pain

As if the complexities of pain management just addressed were not enough, there are the important differences in types of pain, not just differences in patients. Patients with fibromyalgia, chronic fatigue, and small fiber neuropathy suffer from a category of pain known as central intractable pain (CIP)—a type of pain that does not respond to opioids and is, in fact, a type of pain for which the use of opioids has been detrimental [8, 9].

Understanding CIP is vital for diagnosis, and for treatment modalities. Joshi [10] describes the etiology of CIP in terms of brain stimulation due to trauma or injury. NMDA and glutamate are released, and, due to glutamate excitability, glial cells are released. These glial cells are irritated and inflamed, and cytokines release cytotoxins. These cytotoxins are neurotoxins, are pervasive throughout the body, and cause damage to nerves from inflammation. Sensory nerve fibers are specifically targeted. It is important to stress here it is believed that the patient's subjective experience of events as emotionally traumatic in triggering this physiological response that results in cytotoxins' attack on sensory nerve fibers.

There are other variables that can compound and exacerbate this process. There are genes that have been found to be involved in the amplification of pain and may indicate an increased risk of chronic pain development [11]. In addition, there are environmental influences. Previous emotional trauma, sexual abuse, medical influenced trauma, previous stigma from the LGBTQ or other gender related or minority stress inducers has been thought to amplify pain perception. The Substance Abuse and Mental Health Services Administration (SAMSHA) have developed Trauma-informed care education for health care providers for these populations [12].

Treatment is typically a multi-faceted approach to minimize sensitization; there are a number of ways that this can be affected:

1. Prevent the exposure to opioids.

2. Minimize the wind up phenomena. Defined as stimulation of pain nerve fibers to the extent that the fibers are altered and produce neuropathic pain.

3. Setting the expectation for patients prior to painful experiences. Information and education of patients and providers has proven to lower patients' pain scores after surgery.

4. The use of oral Naloxone™ has been on the rise in the recent past due to the research surrounding the stimulation of the midbrain periaqueductal grey (PAG) region. Outputs from the PAG to the medulla reduce pain by activating an endogenous opioidergic pain inhibitory system [13].

5. Lidocaine has been used for over 50 years as a local anesthetic; now it is assisting with less exposure to opioid medications due to its anti-inflammatory and analgesic properties. Postoperative infusions at a low dose have effectively lowered opioid requirements, decreased post-operative nausea, and enhanced the return of bowel function [14].

6. Hormone replacement has been shown to indicate that various hormones regulate the hypothalamic-pituitary-adrenal axis, which, when activated cause persistent pain. Multiple hormones are implicated here, including cortisol and pregnenolone. Dr. Forrest Tennant has developed a protocol for patients who have Ehlers Danlos syndrome and arachnoiditis, which replaces hormones to assist with pain control [15].

7. Dr. Jay Joshi [10] has worked diligently to determine an appropriate plan for individual patients who struggle with CIP, using a treatment plan that relies on ketamine, which has the following benefits:

    - Increase in cerebral blood flow
    - Resetting of the mu receptor
    - Reduction of hypersensitivity
    - Reversal, in some cases, of post-traumatic stress disorder (PTSD)
    - NMDA receptors mediation
    - It serves as a potent neuro-anti-inflammatory agent

Early identification of central pain syndromes prevents the central sensitization and brain reorganization. Functional MRIs show cortical reorganization: psychologic interaction with pain and stress that causes areas in the brain to become hyperactive to a stimulus, including brain mapping and biofeedback [16]. CIP, then, often has its origins in supratentorial factors, and failure to take these factors seriously can result in opioid overuse.

5. The multiple visit patient complex care program

The hospital-based team approach to helping multiple-visit patients has been successful at my suburban hospital for the past 3 years. Recent data indicates the use of individualized care plans by a Complex Care team has helped reduce readmissions by 36%.[1] The goal is to assist the patient to find proper outpatient treatment, so that a readmission to the Emergency Room becomes less necessary. The goals of the care plans include providing appropriate symptom management, as well as reducing the opioids that are prescribed during the Emergency Room visit, and at discharge. Other techniques include giving a welcome letter to a patient that frequently uses the Emergency Room. The goals of the letter are to (1) alert patients to the program; (2) introduce the Complex Care team; (3) offer to help patients obtain a primary care physician; and in accordance with the Center for Disease Control Guidelines; (4) state clearly that we will not always treat their pain with opioids, but will use a multimodal approach when they present for treatment. These specific strategies have reduced the readmission rate by 60–70% during a more specific period of study.

Identification and diagnosis is paramount to optimizing treatment strategies and symptom management. Patients who frequent the Emergency Room can be misunderstood with characteristics that are not always identified early in their pain treatment. This can place the patient at risk for over-medication syndromes, over-utilization of the healthcare system, and developing central sensitization.

Retrospectively, identification of complex patients who have symptoms that correlate to those identified as CIP has been ongoing. Recognizing CIP has resulted in revised treatment plans for patients. Case Study 4 describes one such instance of the importance of recognizing CIP.

Case Study 4

A patient experienced a significant traumatic event when she was young. She developed low back pain and abdominal pain, although the imaging for both were not significant enough to pinpoint the cause for the pain. She had multiple medical procedures and work-ups, and because she complained of severe pain even after other medications, opioids were begun. Over the years, the dosages were increased, but they were not effective. The pain continued despite the subsequent overuse of the opioids. She eventually had multiple admissions to the hospital without a cause for the pain identified.

After being treated for opioid addiction, the patient was introduced to the concept of ketamine treatment for desensitization for central pain. After a series of ketamine infusions, the central sensitization subsided. The patient was able to use significantly less opioids, with much greater relief of the pain. She has now learned to identify the triggers of her pain exacerbations, and has been able to be active and care for her family.

Informal conversations with colleagues at other institutions suggest that our suburban hospital is not the only facility to have concerns about patients similar to the one described above. Recognizing that many pain patients have a type of central sensitization—chronic pain that is out of control—can both reduce pain that is activated by a physical response to a past stressor—and the repeated exposure to opioids.

The case studies below represent how recognizing the role of CIP in supratentorial pain can reduce reliance upon opioids and subsequent opioid-related addiction problems. Some of the implications found in the cases below include non-opioid pain management, the use of postoperative lidocaine, and desensitization with ketamine. This is consistent with the prevention of opioid exposure as the new paradigm, and the need to implement innovative treatments.

[1]Source: unpublished data from 2015 to 2017 (Delnor Hospital, Geneva, Illinois, USA).

Case Study 5

A patient with significant head pain sought diagnosis for her pain at multiple facilities without a definite diagnosis. All headache abortive efforts failed, and all multimodal management failed to relieve the pain. The patient was placed on intravenous meperidine and over the course of many years, the dosage was raised to a high dose. This was effective for a short time, but then the high dose began to fail in efficacy. Re-interpretation of her pain in terms of CIP etiology has resulted in conversations about stressors in her social life, and a reduction of opioids.

Case Study 6

A patient had a cervical spinal cord stimulator placed, but it failed almost immediately, worsening her pain. Struggles with anxiety and debility have contributed to a clinical diagnosis of depression. Treatment for depression has resulted in less frequent PTSD responses to an earlier-life trauma. As a result, her pain is not managed with less reliance on opioids.

Case Study 7

A patient has progressive neuropathy, although the reason is unclear. Initially she presented with the inability to sit up long enough to go to her primary care physician's office, which suggested significant psychological overlay. Opioids were escalated, and her ability to sit comfortably and walk easily did improve. Care conferences ensued and biopsies, along with neurologic medication were used without improvement. Finally, the recognition that CIP might, at least in part, have had a role in the patient's symptoms resulted in fewer symptoms and a consequent reduction of opioids.

6. Conclusion and recommendations

The management of pain by health care providers and pain specialists has a new contour: identify the patients with CIP in a timely manner, then identify treatments and methods to find sustained relief with limited or no use of opioids.

A patient's previous history of PTSD, anxiety (general anxiety disorder, post-partum depression, etc.), chronic pain, or substance use disorder matters when it comes to differential diagnoses. It is vital that health care providers realize the ramifications of co-existing psychological and neurologic impact when planning for surgery or other pain-producing procedures.

What might be routine and typical surgery/procedure from the perspective of a surgeon could be different to the brain, neurotransmitters, and the other aspects of a patient's neuroanatomy. It is crucial that patients' prior history be considered, and a plan put in place to assist the patient in coping. Pre-surgical education and planning, along with collaboration between anesthesia or social work colleagues can have a long-term positive effect. It may be beneficial to place a temporary nerve block, low dose lidocaine, or bupivacaine (either short acting or long-acting) in order to block the ascending nociceptors from sending the pain signal through the descending pain pathway. The future of pain management must be the prevention of pain pathway activation. This will lower the exposure to opioids and prevent future substance use disorder.

Of note, physical therapy is very beneficial to a large subset of patients. Specialized concepts have been developed by physiatrists' (also called physical medicine and rehabilitation specialists) to assist patients with chronic pain, known as an integrative comprehensive pain management program (CPMP). This program revealed significant improvement through the administration of a battery of observed functional tests (BOFT) to patients with chronic pain who were attending the CPMP [13].

Activity can be the best treatment for most pain. Exercise and stretching of muscles, and desensitization of scar tissue leads to healing. Part of the CPMP is cognitive therapy, psychological, neurological, and pain education. It is clear that improving outcomes in chronic pain management occur when the patient understands the influence the mind and the body play in pain perception.

The FDA and other research opportunities should be supported to continue to find more methods of pain blockade and prevention of pain at the site of surgery. Kaiser Permanente and other hospitals around the United States have been adopting the enhanced recovery after surgery (ERAS) concept. There is a full protocol of management of the patient, but the basic tenet is to block the pain to speed recovery with very little or no opioids.

Lowering opioid exposure is paramount and should be supported and rewarded with funding and research grants. Health care and surgeries with minimal or no opioids are possible now, and need to be utilized immediately. Minimizing opioid exposure is the mandate at this time, there are available options presently, and more research dollars should be committed to new ways to block the perception of pain. Finally, patients should be educated about the options and choose hospitals and providers who utilize the most up-to-date resources.

Education of the next generation of providers needs to be clear in the direction and potential options for preventing disability and preventing overuse syndromes, early identification and the importance of prevention of the central sensitization and CIP.

Acknowledgements

The Northwestern Medicine Delnor Hospital Multiple Visit Complex Care Team has offered immeasurable support for the growth of the program. They have supported the patients, the medical staff, and myself through the challenges of the grass roots beginning of the endeavor.

I acknowledge my mentor, Mary Lyons, and will always remember the strength that came from our weekly west region collaboration. The years we worked in tandem were spectacular. I learned so very much from you and feel honored to have you as my esteemed colleague in pain management.

I have truly appreciated Kim Czaruk, Director, who has supported the pain program and has been an encouragement daily.

I thank and respect the patients who struggle with pain and other debilitating symptoms themselves who have taught me invaluable lessons about listening and learning during my years in pain practice. I seek to pass on the non-text book wisdom they have taught me, and pass on the respect for pain management patients that I feel. I believe in thinking outside of the box, and never saying 'there is nothing else I can do for your pain.'

Conflict of interest

No conflict of interest to declare.

Thanks

Thank you to my family, who have eaten cold food, washed my clothes, shopped for groceries, helped keep the house afloat, assisted with edits, and provided tech support. We are on the same team, and I love each one for your support.

Author details

Pamela Bolyanatz
Northwestern Medicine Delnor Hospital, Geneva, Illinois, USA

*Address all correspondence to: pamela.bolyanatz@nm.org

References

[1] Gaskin DJ, Richard P. Institute of Medicine (US) Committee on Advancing Pain Research, Care, and Education. Appendix C: The economic costs of pain in the United States. In: Relieving Pain in America: A Blueprint for Transforming Prevention, Care, Education, and Research. Washington (DC): National Academies Press (US); 2011. Available from: https://www.ncbi.nlm.nih.gov/books/NBK92521/

[2] Booth BM, Walton MA, Barry KL, Cunningham RM, Chermack ST, Blow FC. Substance use, depression and mental health functioning in patients seeking acute medical care in an inner-city ED. The Journal of Behavioral Health Services & Research. 2011;**38**(3):358-372. DOI: 10.1007/s11414-010-9227-6

[3] Quinones S. Dreamland: The True Tale of America's Opioid Epidemic. New York: Bloomsbury Press; 2015

[4] Ossipov M, Dussor G, Porreca F. Central modulation of pain. The Journal of Clinical Investigation. 2010;**120**(11): 3779. DOI: 10.1172/JC143766

[5] Joseph A. CVS Tightens Restrictions on Opioid Prescriptions in Bid to Stanch Epidemic. 2017. Available from: https://www.statnews.com/2017/09/21/cvs-opioid-prescription-limits/ [Accessed: 30 September 2018]

[6] Hill MV, ML MM, Stucke RS, Barth RJ Jr. Wide variation and excessive dosage of opioid prescriptions for common general surgical procedures. Annals of Surgery. 2017;**265**(4):709-714

[7] Schneiderhan J, Orizondo C. Chronic pain how to approach these 3 common conditions. Clinical Reviews. 2017; **27**(10):38-49

[8] Illinois Health and Hospital Association. Opioid Prescribing Guidelines for Patients in the Emergency Department and Immediate Care Centers. 2018. Available from: https://www.team-iha.org/files/non-gated/quality/opioid-guidelines-longversion.aspx [Accessed: 20 September 2018]

[9] Dowell D, Haegerich TM, Chou R. CDC guideline for prescribing opioids for chronic pain—United States. MMWR—Recommendations and Reports. 2016;**65**(RR-1):1-49. DOI: 10.15585/mmwr.rr6501e1 [Accessed: 21 September 2018]

[10] Joshi J. Chronic Pain Advocacy and Consulting Paper presented to the Midwest Pain Treatment and Education Expo. Chicago, Illinois. 2016. Available from: https://www.youtube.com/watch?v=QshZ_unVDQQ [Accessed: 20 September 2018]

[11] Foulkes T, Wood JN. Pain genes. PLoS Genetics. 2008;**4**(7):e1000086. DOI: https://doi.org/10.1371/journal.pgen.1000086 [Accessed: 20 September 2018]

[12] The Substance Abuse and Mental Health Services Administration. n.d. TIP 57, Trauma informed care (TIC)

[13] Oken J, Schwarz L, Brady S. Outcomes in an interdisciplinary comprehensive pain management program. In: Poster Presented to the 41st Midwest Pain Society Scientific Meeting; Chicago, Illinois. 2017

[14] Ventham N, Kennedy E. Efficacy of intravenous lidocaine for postoperative analgesia following laparoscopic surgery: A meta-analysis. World Journal of Surgery. 2015;**39**:220-2234

[15] Tennant F, Lichota L. Testosterone replacement in chronic pain patients. Practical Pain Management. 2010;**10**(6): 12-15. www.foresttennant.com [Accessed: 15 September 2018]

[16] Amen D. The Most Important Lesson From 83,000 Brain Scans; TED Talk. 2013. Available from: https://www.youtube.com/watch?v=esPRsT-lmw8 [Accessed: 20 September 2018]

Chapter 3

Other Uses of Morphine

Shrenik Ostwal

Abstract

Worldwide many different strong opioids and their formulations are available to control pain. Of which, morphine is considered as global opioid of choice and is widely used to control moderate to severe pain. The World Health Organization (WHO) has recommended morphine as one of the essential drug. Apart from analgesic use, research has proven its effectiveness for relief and treatment of various debilitating and distressing conditions like breathlessness, mucositis (oral and vaginal) and cough. However, its role in diarrhea and opioid substitution therapy (OST) is still nonconfirmatory. This chapter illustrates all available literature supporting effectiveness of morphine in above conditions and its impact on quality of life.

Keywords: morphine, dyspnoea, mucositis, chronic cough,
opioid substitution therapy (OST), diarrhea

1. Introduction

Preparations of the opium poppy *Papaver somniferum* have been used for many hundreds of years to relieve pain. Morphine remains as the gold standard for management of moderate to severe cancer pain. It has a five ringed structure with a characteristic T-shaped three dimensional form essential for activation of the opioid receptor.

Due to its strong affinity to mu receptors and action similar to endorphins, i.e., natural pain killers, morphine has been widely used globally. Apart from its analgesic action, it can be used widely for symptomatic relief of other distressing and debilitating conditions. This chapter depicts all available literature for various other uses of morphine.

2. Dyspnoea

2.1 Introduction

Dyspnoea, also termed as breathlessness, is a common and prevalent source of discomfort in patients with advanced cancer and non-cancer life limiting illnesses. Most people describe it as an uncomfortable sensation or increased work of breathing in terms of air hunger, increased effort, chest tightness, rapid breathing, incomplete exhalation or feeling of suffocation.

The American Thoracic Society defined dyspnoea as "a subjective experience of breathing discomfort that consists of qualitatively distinct sensations that vary in intensity" [1]. This definition highlights key areas where dyspnoea can be measured, suggesting that dyspnoea is not merely a single sensation but a shared experience with physical and affective components. This is similar to concept of total pain or total suffering which constitutes other domains like psychological, social, spiritual and environmental.

The prevalence of dyspnoea varies according to disease primary site and stage of illness. Studies by Muers and Round [2]; Smith et al. [3] reported prevalence of dyspnoea in 75–87% patients with primary lung cancer. While, a systematic review by Solano et al. [4] reported dyspnoea prevalence of: 90–95% in patients with chronic obstructive pulmonary disease (COPD), 60–88% in patients with heart disease, 11–62% in patients with AIDS and 11–62% in patients with renal disease. COPD and chronic heart failure (CHF) constitutes major non-cancer causes of dyspnoea in patients [5, 6].

Dyspnoea due to its prevalence and associated suffering poses a significant burden to patients and caregivers, hence severely affecting quality of life.

2.2 Pathophysiology of dyspnoea

Normally during unconscious activity, respiration is managed by clusters of neurons in the medulla. They receive afferent input from several types of mechanoreceptors in respiratory muscles, airways, and lung parenchyma and chemoreceptors in aortic and carotid bodies and the medulla. Motor commands from the medulla or motor cortex by means of the medulla descend to respiratory muscles through efferent motor neurons [7, 8].

Differential diagnosis for dyspnoea in advanced cancer can be: (**Table 1**).

2.3 Opioids in breathlessness

The primary site of action of opioids in breathlessness is through medulla oblongata, although various mechanisms may be involved on effect on perception of breathlessness. **Box 1** suggests various mechanisms by which morphine acts on breathlessness [1].

- Analgesia—reduction of pain induced respiratory drive.
- Anxiolytic effects.
- Reduce minute ventilation.
- Cortical sedation (suppression of respiratory awareness).
- Alteration of neurotransmission within medullary respiratory center.
- Reduce central sensitivity and response to hypercarbia or hypoxia.
- Decreased metabolic rate and ventilatory requirements—decrease in O_2 consumption.
- Vasodilatation and improved cardiac functions.

Box 1.
Mechanism by which morphine reduces perception of breathlessness. Source: Adapted from American Thoracic Society guidelines on dyspnoea 2012.

A study by Mahler et al. [9] in 2009 demonstrated threefold increase in beta endorphin levels in 17 COPD patients when compared from rest to end exercise. Patients were randomized to receive either normal saline or 10 mg of intravenous naloxone. Authors found significantly higher peak ratings and regression slope of breathlessness with naloxone as compared to normal saline. This study high-lighten role of endogenous opioids in dyspnoea modification in COPD patients.

Research has demonstrated role of oral morphine in breathlessness. However dosing schedule varies according to underlying condition. **Box 2** depicts morphine dosing recommendations for breathlessness [10]:

- Opioids should be started when disabling dyspnoea persists despite maximal Management of underlying condition.
- Check for renal, hepatic, pulmonary function, current and past opioid use.
- Prescribe laxatives and other supportive medications.
- Adopt policy of "Start Low and Go Slow" while titrating morphine dosage.
- Titrate morphine dose (up to 25–50% of dose for continued mild to moderate dyspnoea; and by up to 50–100% of dose for continued moderate to severe dyspnoea) every weekly over 4 weeks until lowest effective dose is found.
- Start with 2.5–5 mg/4 h. PO or 1–2.5 mg/4 h. SC of morphine in opioid naive patients.
- For patients already prescribed morphine for pain, increase regular dose by 25–30%.
- Consider long acting twice daily morphine dosing in patients with stable regular dose.
- Consider 1/6th of regular dose prn for episodic breathlessness.

Box 2.
Morphine dosing recommendations for breathlessness. Source: Adapted and developed from best practice for managing breathlessness in palliative care.

Malignant causes	Non-malignant causes
Lung cancer/metastases to lung	COPD/interstitial lung disease
Pleural effusion/pericardial effusion/ascites	Bronchiectasis
Superior vena caval obstruction	Congestive heart failure
Pulmonary embolism	Arrhythmias
Pulmonary edema	Motor neuron diseases
Major airway obstruction	Muscular dystrophy
Lymphangitis carcinomatosis	Anaemia
Chest wall infiltration	Acidosis
Radiation induced pulmonary fibrosis	Anxiety/panic attacks

Table 1.
Causes of dyspnoea.

2.3.1 Morphine for breathlessness in cancer patients

There is good evidence for role of opioids in breathlessness [1, 5, 11–20]. Most of studies illustrated beneficial effect of morphine in breathlessness in cancer patients. Out of eight studies which evaluated effect of morphine in cancer related dyspnoea, seven were randomized controlled, double blind trials [21]. Another study by Clemens et al. [22], a non-randomized prospective study in advanced terminal cancer patients with dyspnoea, reported beneficial effect of morphine in reducing intensity of dyspnoea when compared with oxygen. While, Charles et al. [23] also reported similar and rapid improvement in breathlessness with use of nebulised hydromorphone. Studies by Bruera et al. [15] and Mazocato et al. [24] compared role of subcutaneous morphine with placebo in patients with primary lung cancer or lung metastases, showing a significant decrease in breathlessness intensity on visual analogue scale (VAS) after 45 min of intervention when treated with morphine. This was supported by a meta-analysis by Ben-Aharon et al. [10] in patients with cancer related dyspnoea. Authors found positive effect of opioids in reducing breathlessness.

Another two studies by Davis et al. (1996) and Grimbert et al. [25] reported no significant improvement in VAS scores even after 60 min of intervention with nebulized morphine when compared with placebo, i.e., nebulised saline. In one study Bruera et al. [15] compared effect of subcutaneous morphine with nebulised morphine in lung primary patients, reporting no significant difference in dyspnoea intensity. However, this study reported patient's preference with nebulised morphine. Lastly, Allard et al. [26] found no significant differences in VAS score with 25 or 50% increments in morphine dosages.

2.3.2 Morphine for breathlessness in COPD patients

A systemic review and meta-analysis by Jennings et al., comparing opioids with placebo for the treatment of dyspnoea [21] showed out of 18 randomized controlled trials (RCT) involved, nine trials reported patients receiving either oral opioids ($n = 8$) or subcutaneous morphine ($n = 1$). Such patients experienced significant beneficial effect with parenteral opioids on reducing dyspnoea when compared with placebo (meanΔ: −0.40; CI: −0.32 to −0.17). However, exercise was used as provoking stimulus to dyspnoea in eight of these nine studies, whereas only one study could examine patients with dyspnoea at rest.

Another randomized, double blind, placebo-controlled crossover trial by Abernethy et al. [27] compared 4 days of 20 mg oral sustained-release morphine with 4 days of oral placebo. Thirty-eight (87.5%) participants who were opioid naive and had dyspnoea at rest in spite of optimal therapy for their underlying condition (mainly patients with COPD) completed the trial. Patients on morphine experienced significant improvements (i.e., less dyspnoea and improved sleep) on VAS scale. Hence, authors concluded that "sustained release, oral morphine at low dosage provides significant symptomatic improvement in refractory dyspnoea in the community setting."

2.3.3 Morphine for breathlessness in heart failure patients

Only few published studies have demonstrated positive outcomes with use of morphine in CHF related dyspnoea. In a pilot study by Johnson et al. [28] aimed to measure effect of oral morphine on breathlessness in patients with CHF, authors found a significant decrease in median breathlessness in those who received 5 mg of oral morphine four times a day ($p = 0.022$), whereas no change was observed in patients treated with placebo.

Oxberry et al. [29] conducted a crossover RCT on 35 patients diagnosed with CHF (New York Heart Association Grade III–IV) comparing 4 days of morphine (5 mg four times daily), oxycodone (2.5 mg four times daily) and placebo followed by a washout period of 3 days. Patients were followed up for 3 months. Authors found a significant improvement in composite breathlessness in opioid group as compared to placebo ($p = 0.017$). However they did not find any statistically significant difference in breathlessness improvement in either intervention group. Hence, authors concluded need for long term trials to establish effectiveness of opioids.

Before stating opioids for dyspnoea in CHF patients, all possible etio-pathological causes should be taken into consideration. Non-pharmacological treatment options—salt and fluid restriction, diet modification, appropriate exercise training and weight reduction strategies, etc., should be used first. Pharmacological therapy with angiotensin converting enzyme (ACE) inhibitors, angiotensin receptor blockers (ARB), beta blockers, diuretics, digoxin and implant devices should be optimally considered. Other possible causes like anaemia and pleural effusion should be taken care of.

2.3.4 Morphine for breathlessness in other conditions

A recent double blind study by Shohrati et al. [30] on 40 patients presented with dyspnoea due to mustard gas induced bronchiolitis obliterans reported effectiveness of nebulised morphine (1 mg diluted in 4 cc normal saline). Patients experienced improvements in dyspnoea VAS score, cough, night time awakenings both due to dyspnoea and cough, heart rate, respiratory rate and overall quality of life.

A phase I clinical trial on six patients with interstitial lung disease (ILD) by Matsuda et al. [31] comparing two different doses of subcutaneous morphine injection demonstrated a tolerable dose of 2 mg to alleviate dyspnoea. However due to small sample size, results could not be reciprocated to general population and need for larger trials were recommended. On the other hand, Harris-Eze et al. [32] does not found any significant difference in exercise capacity and dyspnoea score in ILD patients treated with either 2.5 or 5 mg of nebulised morphine. This was supported by Cochrane review by Polosa et al. [33].

A single arm study of six patients with terminal amyotrophic lateral sclerosis (ALS) by Clemens et al. [22] showed effectiveness of morphine in reducing dyspnoea. Authors found a significant difference in respiratory rate and dyspnoea intensity at 120 min after morphine administration.

3. Role of morphine in mucositis

Mucositis refers to erythematous, erosive and ulcerative lesion of mucosa observed in patients with cancer treated with chemotherapy and/or radiotherapy to fields involving areas of body. Accordingly it may involve oral cavity, gastrointestinal tract, vaginal mucosa or other areas. Hence, manifesting as burning pain in mouth, diarrhea, vaginitis, etc. Elting et al. [34] observed chemotherapy-induced mucositis in 303 out of 599 patients (51%). Oral mucositis was developed in 22% cycles while gastrointestinal (GI) mucositis in 7% cycles.

3.1 Pathophysiology of mucositis

The five-stage model depicts various steps involved in pathogenesis of mucositis. Stages involved are [35]:

1. Stage of initiation of tissue injury

2. Stage of signaling through up regulation of inflammation *via* generation of messenger signals

3. Stage of amplification

4. Stage of ulceration and inflammation

5. Stage of healing

3.2 Morphine and oral mucositis

Oral mucositis poses a significant source of pain and distress to patients receiving chemotherapy or radiotherapy to head and neck area. It often manifests as burning pain, ulcers, erythematous lesions in mouth complicated by secondary infections—bacterial/fungal/viral. It significantly affects nutritional intake, oral hygiene and overall quality of life. Infections associated with oral mucositis may pose life-threatening conditions. Adequate oral hygiene and treatment of underlying cause helps to relieve symptoms and distress in patients [36, 37].

Various combination of local measures helps to take care of mucositis-related complications. Research has shown effectiveness of morphine gargles either alone (morphine rinse) or in combination with antacid, lignocaine viscous and dextromethorphan (magic mouth wash), in relieving pain and symptoms related to mucositis. A mini review by Dutta et al. [38] compared six studies using morphine as oral rinse. All studies showed satisfactory result in terms of pain control, mouth opening and patient preferences. This is supported by other studies which proved efficacy of morphine gargles [36, 37, 39–44].

3.3 Morphine and vaginal mucositis

Vaginitis, also known as vaginal mucositis is an acute inflammation with erythema and erosion of vaginal mucosa leading to severe vaginal pain, per vaginal discharge and/or associated complications. It is commonly seen in patients with local infection or as a part of systemic infection, as a complication to radiotherapy to local areas or chemotherapy, recto-vaginal fistula, trauma, etc. Morphine, similar to its role in oral mucositis can be considered for vaginal mucositis. A case reported by Ostwal et al. [45] showed efficacy of morphine when combined with vaginal douche (magic vaginal douche—metronidazole, normal saline, povidone iodine solution, lignocaine viscous with 20 mg crushed tab morphine) in relief from symptoms of vaginal mucositis. However RCTs are not available and are required to prove its clinical efficacy.

4. Role of morphine in chronic cough

4.1 Introduction

Cough is found to be prevalent in around 65% patients with lung cancer [46] and 70% patients with COPD [47, 48]. Persistent or chronic cough can have various physical complications like musculoskeletal pain over chest wall, rib fracture, bowel and bladder incontinence, disturbed sleep and feeling of exhaustion. Patients usually experience psychological impacts, social isolation and decreased quality of life [48].

Cough reflex is regulated by vagal afferent pathways, nucleus tractus solitarius (NTS) in brainstem, and cough center in cerebral cortex. Common underlying patho-physiological causes for cough includes: (i) infection; (ii) lung cancer or secondary metastases to lung/pleura/mediastinum/pericardium/blood vessels; (iii) COPD, ILD, bronchiectasis; (iv) aspiration; (v) asthma/bronchospasm; (vi) esophageal reflux; (vii) tracheo-esophageal fistula; (viii) radiotherapy or chemotherapy induced pulmonary fibrosis; (ix) ACE inhibitors; (x) pulmonary edema/left ventricular failure, etc. Timely and proper assessment of cough with removal of underlying cause can decrease distress and improve patients' quality of life.

4.2 Morphine and cough

Research work by Kamei [49] showed involvement of mu opioid receptors in production of cough. Very limited studies are available for use of morphine on chronic cough [47, 50–56]. Strongest evidence for effectiveness of morphine in chronic cough was shown in a double blind placebo controlled trial by Morice et al. [57]. Twenty seven patients with chronic persistent cough were assigned to 4 weeks of slow release morphine sulfate (5 mg twice daily escalated to 10 mg twice daily) matched correspondingly with placebo. A significant improvement of 3.2 points over baseline, and 40% rapid reduction in cough frequency and severity was observed in slow release morphine group ($p < 0.01$). Dose comparison over 3 month period between 5 and 10 mg did not showed any significant difference, helping to conclude study with daily dose recommendation of slow release morphine sulfate from 5 to 10 mg twice daily.

5. Role of morphine in diarrhea

Diarrhea has been defined as "passage of ≥3 loose or watery bowel movements per day or passage of ≥200 g of stool per day based on typical diet." Diarrhea can be acute (<14 days), persistent (>14 days but <30 days) or chronic (>30 days) based on its duration. Diarrhea poses a common and significant problem in patients with cancer. It may be due to either local infection, as a part of systemic inflammation/infection, as a complication to radiotherapy or chemotherapy [58], etc.

Mechanism for diarrhea can be attributed to increased intestinal motility [59, 60]. Hence drugs which act to decrease intestinal motility are found to be helpful in treatment. Morphine and other opiates (loperamide, diphenoxylate, codeine) act on intestinal mu-receptors and slow intestinal transit time, thus increasing net absorption [61, 62]. Though constipation is commonly seen as a side effect with morphine use, research considering use of this side effect to treat diarrhea has not been done. Clinical Practice guidelines by European Society for Medical Oncology (ESMO) has documented role of tincture of opium like morphine (10 mg/mL morphine) in treatment with diarrhea as an alternative to loperamide. The recommended dose of tincture morphine is 10–15 drops in water every 3–4 h [58, 63, 64]. Till date robust studies supporting this has not been available.

6. Morphine and opioid substitution therapy (OST)

Morphine has been known for its potential effect in analgesia since last few decades. However, it is also known for its potential to cause addiction and dependence. Opium, derived naturally from poppy plant is widely used for addiction. Opioid substitution therapy (OST) is an evidence-based intervention for opiate dependent persons that replaces illicit drug use with medically prescribed, orally administered opiates such as buprenorphine and methadone. OST reduces HIV risk behaviors and harms associated with injecting (such as abscesses, septicemia and endocarditis), overdose and participation in criminal activity, thereby improving the quality of life and health of injecting drug users (IDUs).

Work by Hämmig et al. [65] showed that slow release oral morphine (SROM) preparations can be used as OST for heroin addicted patients. Authors found higher treatment satisfaction, fewer cravings for drug and less mental stress with SROM. Cochrane review by Ferri et al. [65] found only three randomized controlled trials which included SROM for OST. Out of three, only two studies suggested possible role of SROM formulations; while remaining study was associated with adverse events like depressive symptoms [65–70]. Hence authors concluded for necessity of more robust and clinically controlled trials.

7. Conclusion

Morphine, a potent and strong opioid, has shown its efficacy in relieving variety of distressing symptoms. Research has documented role of low dose morphine for treatment and relief from conditions like chronic, refractory breathlessness, cough, mucositis (oral/vaginal). However, more robust studies are required to establish its clinical efficacy in diarrhea and opioid substitution therapy.

Conflicts of interest

None.

Author details

Shrenik Ostwal
Narayana Super Speciality Hospital, Howrah, West Bengal, India

*Address all correspondence to: drshrenikostwal@gmail.com

References

[1] Parshall MB et al. An official American thoracic society statement: Update on the mechanisms, assessment, and management of dyspnoea. American Journal of Respiratory and Critical Care Medicine. 2012;**185**(4):435-452

[2] Muers MF, Round CE. Palliation of symptoms in non-small cell lung cancer: A study by the Yorkshire Regional Cancer Organisation thoracic group. Thorax. 1993;**48**(4):339-343

[3] Smith EL et al. Dyspnea, anxiety, body consciousness, and quality of life in patients with lung cancer. Journal of Pain and Symptom Management. 2001;**21**(4):323-329

[4] Solano JP, Gomes B, Higginson IJ. A comparison of symptom prevalence in far advanced cancer, AIDS, heart disease, chronic obstructive pulmonary disease and renal disease. Journal of Pain and Symptom Management. 2006;**31**(1):58-69

[5] Reuben DB, Mor V. Dyspnea in terminally ill cancer patients. Chest. 1986;**89**(2):234-236

[6] Higginson I, McCarthy M. Measuring symptoms in terminal cancer: Are pain and dyspnoea controlled? Journal of the Royal Society of Medicine. 1989;**82**(5):264-267

[7] Mahler DA, O'Donnell DE. Recent advances in dyspnea. Chest. 2015;**147**(1):232-241

[8] Nishino T. Dyspnoea: Underlying mechanisms and treatment. British Journal of Anaesthesia. 2011;**106**(4):463-474

[9] Mahler DA et al. Endogenous opioids modify dyspnoea during treadmill exercise in patients with COPD. The European Respiratory Journal. 2009;**33**(4):771-777

[10] Ben-Aharon I, Gafter-Gvili A, Leibovici L, Stemmer SM. Interventions for alleviating cancer-related dyspnea: A systematic review. Journal of Clinical Oncology. 2008;**26**(14):2396-2404

[11] Cabezón-Gutiérrez L, Khosravi-Shahi P, Custodio-Cabello S, Muñiz-González F, Cano-Aguirre M d P, Alonso-Viteri S. Opioids for management of episodic breathlessness or dyspnea in patients with advanced disease. Supportive Care in Cancer. 2016;**24**(9):4045-4055

[12] Currow D et al. A pragmatic, phase III, multisite, double-blind, placebo-controlled, parallel-arm, dose increment randomised trial of regular, low-dose extended-release morphine for chronic breathlessness: Breathlessness, exertion and morphine sulfate (BEAMS) study protocol On behalf of the Australian National Palliative Care Clinical Studies Collaborative (PaCCSC). BMJ Open. 2017;**7**:18-100

[13] Barnes H, McDonald J, Smallwood N, Manser R. Opioids for the palliation of refractory breathlessness in adults with advanced disease and terminal illness. Cochrane Database of Systematic Reviews. 31 Mar 2016;**3**:CD011008. DOI: 10.1002/14651858.CD011008.pub2

[14] Afolabi TM, Nahata MC, Pai V. Nebulized opioids for the palliation of dyspnea in terminally ill patients. American Journal of Health-System Pharmacy. 2017;**74**(14):1053-1061

[15] Bruera E, Macmillan K, Pither J, MacDonald RN. Effects of morphine on the dyspnea of terminal cancer patients. Journal of Pain and Symptom Management. 1990;**5**(6):341-344

[16] Kloke M, Cherny N. Treatment of dyspnoea in advanced cancer patients: ESMO Clinical Practice Guidelines. Annals of Oncology. 2015;**26**(5):69-73

[17] Thomas JR, von Gunten CF. Clinical management of dyspnoea. The Lancet Oncology. 2002;**3**(4):223-228

[18] Ben-Aharon I, Gafter-Gvili A, Leibovici L, Stemmer SM. Interventions for alleviating cancer-related dyspnea: A systematic review and meta-analysis. Acta Oncologica. 2012;**51**(8):996-1008

[19] Mahler DA. Opioids for refractory dyspnea. Expert Review of Respiratory Medicine. 2013;**7**(2):123-135

[20] Tian C, Wang JY, Wang ML, Jiang B, Zhang LL, Liu F. Morphine versus methylprednisolone or aminophylline for relieving dyspnea in patients with advanced cancer in China: A retrospective study. Springerplus. 2016;**5**(1):1945

[21] Jennings A-L, Davies AN, Higgins JPT, Gibbs JSR, Broadley KE. A systematic review of the use of opioids in the management of dyspnoea. Thorax. 2002;**57**(11):939-944

[22] Clemens KE, Quednau I, Klaschik E. Is there a higher risk of respiratory depression in opioid-naïve palliative care patients during symptomatic therapy of dyspnea with strong opioids? Journal of Palliative Medicine. 2008;**11**(2):204-216

[23] Charles MA, Reymond L, Israel F. Relief of incident dyspnea in palliative cancer patients: A pilot, randomized, controlled trial comparing nebulized hydromorphone, systemic hydromorphone, and nebulized saline. Journal of Pain and Symptom Management. 2008;**36**(1):29-38

[24] Mazzocato C, Buclin T, Rapin CH. The effects of morphine on dyspnea and ventilatory function in elderly patients with advanced cancer: A randomized double-blind controlled trial. Annals of Oncology: Official Journal of the European Society for Medical Oncology/ESMO. 1999;**10**(12):1511-1514

[25] Grimbert D et al. Dyspnea and morphine aerosols in the palliative care of lung cancer. Revue des Maladies Respiratoires. 2004;**21**(6):1091-1097

[26] Schwartzman RJ, Patel M, Grothusen JR, Alexander GM. Efficacy of 5-day continuous lidocaine infusion for the treatment of refractory complex regional pain syndrome. Pain Medicine. 2009;**10**(2):401-412

[27] Abernethy AP, Currow DC, Frith P, Fazekas BS, McHugh A, Bui C. Randomised, double blind, placebo controlled crossover trial of sustained release morphine for the management of refractory dyspnoea. BMJ [British Medical Journal]. 2003;**327**(7414):523-528

[28] Johnson MJ, Mcdonagh TA, Harkness A, Mckay SE, Dargie HJ, Infirmary GR. Morphine for the relief of breathlessness in patients with chronic heart failure—A pilot study. The European Journal of Heart Failure. 2002;**4**:753-756

[29] Oxberry SG, Bland JM, Clark AL, Cleland JG, Johnson MJ. Repeat dose opioids may be effective for breathlessness in chronic heart failure if given for long enough. Journal of Palliative Medicine. 2013;**16**(3):250-255

[30] Shohrati M, Ghanei M, Harandi AA, Foroghi S, Harandi AA. Effect of nebulized morphine on dyspnea of mustard gas-exposed patients: A double-blind randomized clinical trial study. Pulmonary medicine. 2012;**2012**:1-6

[31] Matsuda Y et al. Low-dose morphine for dyspnea in terminally ill patients with idiopathic interstitial pneumonias. Journal of Palliative Medicine. 2017;**20**(8):879-883

[32] Harris-Eze AO, Sridhar G, Clemens RE, Zintel TA, Gallagher CG, Marciniuk DD. Low-dose nebulized morphine

does not improve exercise in interstitial lung disease. American Journal of Respiratory and Critical Care Medicine. 1995;**152**(6):1940-1945

[33] Polosa R, Simidchiev A, Walters EH. Nebulised morphine for severe interstitial lung disease. Cochrane Database of Systematic Reviews. 2002;**3**:CD002872

[34] Elting LS, Cooksley C, Chambers M, Cantor SB, Manzullo E, Rubenstein EB. The burdens of cancer therapy: Clinical and economic outcomes of chemotherapy-induced mucositis. Cancer. 2003;**98**(7):1531-1539

[35] Lalla RV, Sonis ST, Peterson DE. Management of oral mucositis in patients who have cancer. Dental Clinics of North America. 2008;**52**(1):61-77

[36] Lalla RV, Bowen J, Barasch A, et al. MASCC/ISOO Clinical Practice Guidelines for the management of mucositis secondary to cancer therapy. Cancer. 2014;**120**(10):1453-1461

[37] Joanna Briggs Institute. Prevention and treatment of oral mucositis in cancer patients. Best Practice. 1998;**2**(3):1-6

[38] Dutta K, Garg R, Garg R. Palliative medicine and hospice care morphine mouthwash in oral mucositis: A mini review. The American Journal of Hospice & Palliative Care. 2016;**2**(2):26-29

[39] Saroja G, Devi PS, Namrata R. Oral morphine solution as an oral rinse or mouth gargle for mucositis pain. Indian Journal of Palliative Care. 2010;**16**(1):54-55

[40] Sarvizadeh M, Hemati S, Meidani M, Ashouri M, Roayaei M, Shahsanai A. Morphine mouthwash for the management of oral mucositis in patients with head and neck cancer. Advanced Biomedical Research. 2015;**4**(1):44

[41] Saunders DP et al. Systematic review of antimicrobials, mucosal coating agents, anesthetics, and analgesics for the management of oral mucositis in cancer patients. Supportive Care in Cancer. 2013;**21**(11):3191-3207

[42] Quinn B. Efficacy of a supersaturated calcium phosphate oral rinse for the prevention and treatment of oral mucositis in patients receiving high-dose cancer therapy: A review of current data. European Journal of Cancer Care. 2013;**22**(5):564-579

[43] Cerchietti LCA et al. Effect of topical morphine for mucositis-associated pain following concomitant chemoradiotherapy for head and neck carcinoma. Cancer. 2002;**95**(10):2230-2236

[44] Chan A, Ignoffo RJ. Survey of topical oral solutions for the treatment of chemo-induced oral mucositis. Journal of Oncology Pharmacy Practice. 2005;**11**(4):139-143

[45] Anandi Q, Ostwal S, Patel H, Sanghavi P. Magic vaginal douche for severe vaginal mucositis: A case-based approach. International Journal of Palliative Nursing. 2018;**1**(1):17-18

[46] Kvale PA. Chronic cough due to lung tumors ACCP evidence-based clinical practice guidelines. Chest. Jan 2006;**129**(1 Suppl):147S-153S. DOI: 10.1378/chest.129.1_suppl.147S

[47] Molassiotis A et al. Clinical expert guidelines for the management of cough in lung cancer: Report of a UK task group on cough. Cough. 2010;**6**(1):9

[48] Molassiotis A, Bailey C, Caress A, Tan JY. Interventions for cough in cancer. Cochrane Database of Systematic Reviews. 2010;**9**: CD007881

[49] Kamei J. Role of opioidergic and serotonergic mechanisms in cough and

antitussives. Pulmonary Pharmacology. 1996;**9**(5-6):349-356

[50] Dudgeon DJ. Managing dyspnea and cough. Hematology/ Oncology Clinics of North America. 2002;**16**(3):557-577

[51] An HJ, Kim I-K, Lee JE, Kang Y-J, Kim CH, Kim H-K. Nebulized morphine for intractable cough in advanced cancer: Two case reports. Journal of Palliative Medicine. 2015;**18**(3):278-281

[52] Gibson P, Wang G, McGarvey L, Vertigan AE, Altman KW, Birring SS. Treatment of unexplained chronic cough chest guideline and expert panel report. Chest. 2016;**149**(1):27-44

[53] Wee B et al. Management of chronic cough in patients receiving palliative care: Review of evidence and recommendations by a task group of the Association for Palliative Medicine of Great Britain and Ireland. Palliative Medicine. 2012;**26**(6):780-787

[54] Stein WM, Min YK. Nebulized morphine for paroxysmal cough and dyspnea in a nursing home resident with metastatic cancer. American Journal of Hospice and Palliative Medicine. 1997;**14**(2):52-56

[55] Borja-Cacho D, Matthews J. NIH public access. Nano. 2008;**6**(9):2166-2171

[56] Badri H, Satia I, Woodcock A, Smith J. The use of low dose morphine for the management of chronic cough in a tertiary cough clinic background: Objective: Methods. American Journal of Respiratory and Critical Care Medicine. 2015;**191**:A4117

[57] Morice AH et al. Opiate therapy in chronic cough. American Journal of Respiratory and Critical Care Medicine. 2007;**175**(4):312-315

[58] Bush SH et al. Diarrhoea in adult cancer patients: ESMO Clinical Practice Guidelines. Annals of Oncology. 2018;**29**(4):iv126-iv142

[59] Porreca F, Heyman JS, Mosberg HI, Omnaas JR, Vaught JL. Role of mu and delta receptors in the supraspinal and spinal analgesic effects of [D-Pen2, D-Pen5] enkephalin in the mouse. The Journal of Pharmacology and Experimental Therapeutics. 1987;**241**(2):393-400

[60] Wood JD, Galligan JJ. Function of opioids in the enteric nervous system. Neurogastroenterology and Motility. 2004;**16**(s2):17-28

[61] Kaufman PN et al. Role of opiate receptors in the regulation of colonic transit. Gastroenterology. 1988;**94**:1351-1356

[62] Sternini C, Patierno S, Selmer I-S, Kirchgessner A. The opioid system in the gastrointestinal tract. Neurogastroenterology and Motility. 2004;**16**(s2):3-16

[63] Cherny NI. Evaluation and management of treatment-related diarrhea in patients with advanced cancer: A review. Journal of Pain and Symptom Management. 2008;**36**(4):413-423

[64] Schiller LR, Pardi DS, Sellin JH. Chronic diarrhea: Diagnosis and management. Clinical Gastroenterology and Hepatology. 2017;**15**(2):182-193

[65] Hämmig R et al. Safety and tolerability of slow-release oral morphine versus methadone in the treatment of opioid dependence. Journal of Substance Abuse Treatment. 2014;**47**(4):275-281

[66] Ferri M, Minozzi S, Bo A, Amato L. Slow-release oral morphine as maintenance therapy for opioid

dependence. Cochrane Database of Systematic Reviews. 2013;**6**:CD009879. DOI: 10.1002/14651858.CD009879.pub2

[67] Eder H, Jagsch R, Kraigher D, Primorac A, Ebner N, Fischer G. Comparative study of the effectiveness of slow-release morphine and methadone for opioid maintenance therapy. Addiction. 2005;**100**(8):1101-1109

[68] Kraigher D et al. Use of slow-release oral morphine for the treatment of opioid dependence. European Addiction Research. 2005;**11**(3):145-151

[69] Giacomuzzi S, Kemmler G, Ertl M, Riemer Y. Opioid addicts at admission vs. slow-release oral morphine, methadone, and sublingual buprenorphine maintenance treatment participants. Substance Use & Misuse. 2006;**41**(2):223-244

[70] Beck T et al. Maintenance treatment for opioid dependence with slow-release oral morphine: A randomized cross-over, non-inferiority study versus methadone. Addiction. 2013;**109**:617-626

Section 3

Pathophysiology and Therapeutic Strategies for Opioid Addiction

Chapter 4

Role of Glucocorticoid Receptor in the Relation between Stress and Opiate Addiction

Javier Navarro-Zaragoza, María Victoria Milanés and María Luisa Laorden

Abstract

Stressful situations can result in relapse in dependent or abstinent causing reinstatement of drug-seeking. In fact, it has been suggested that activation of the brain stress system results in glucocorticoid release that affects the dopaminergic pathways. Also, the noradrenergic system innervates the extrahypothalamic BSS from the nucleus of tractus solitarius (NTS), resulting in a feedforward loop between the corticotropin-releasing factor (CRF) and noradrenaline (NA) crucial in drug addiction and relapses. Glucocorticoids interact with two receptors: mineralocorticoid receptor (MR) and glucocorticoid receptor (GR) which bind to a GRE site located in tyrosine hydroxylase (TH), resulting in the upregulation of TH synthesis and, finally, increasing dopamine (DA) release in the nucleus accumbens. TH upregulation depends on the phosphorylation of serine 31 and/or serine 40. Previous research has shown that protein kinase C (PKC) activates extracellular signal-regulated kinase (ERK) pathway and in turn phosphorylates serine 31 in the NTS. Besides, cAMP response element binding protein (CREB) is regulated by PKA and PKC. The results shown after pretreating morphine-withdrawn rats with mifepristone and spironolactone (GR and MR antagonists, respectively) suggest that glucocorticoids have a prominent role in addiction because GR would activate ERK and CREB in the NTS, phosphorylating serine 31 and activating TH and indeed noradrenergic release in the paraventricular nucleus (PVN).

Keywords: glucocorticoids, stress, addiction, brain stress system, noradrenergic system, TH, ERK, CREB

1. Introduction

Drug addiction is a chronic disease characterized by recurrence of its signs: drug-seeking and drug-taking behavior, loss of control and impulsivity in consumption, and emergence of a negative state when the access to the drug is not possible [1]. Besides, drug relapse is very often even months and years after withdrawal [2].

Drug addiction has been described as a three-phase disease: During phase 1, drug- seeking behavior is exacerbated and it courses with sensibilization of dopaminergic system, altogether with an associative learning from environment [3]. Phase 2 consists of positive reinforcement pathway downregulation [4]. Finally, phase 3 is characterized by a negative emotional state and by an enhanced craving, which facilitates relapse to drug addiction [5]. Summarizing, individuals experience positive reinforcement in early stages of addiction when they consume drugs of abuse, but after several intakes, they continue that consumption only to avoid the negative state that appears during withdrawal [2, 6].

Previous research has described the importance of different neurotransmitters and neuronal systems in the distinct phases of addiction, being dopaminergic system the main responsible of positive reinforcement [7–10]. Differently, noradrenergic system and brain stress system activities are increased during drug dependence [11].

It is well known that dopaminergic system innervates the prefrontal cortex (PFC) and the nucleus accumbens (NAc), where consumption of major drugs of abuse produces dopamine (DA) release, what is attributed to be behind the development of drug addiction due to its positive reinforcement properties. In contrast, noradrenergic system is mainly related with the negative state that emerges when there is drug withdrawal. It has been shown that noradrenergic innervation from nucleus of tractus solitarius (NTS) to the paraventricular nucleus (PVN) is involved in drug-seeking and in the negative reinforcement produced by morphine withdrawal [12, 13]. Moreover, the existence of a loop between noradrenaline (NA) and corticotropin-releasing factor (CRF) has been described where the enhancement of NA system would result in the enhancement of CRF release (feedforward) and vice versa [14].

On the other hand, many pathways are involved in drug addiction resulting in intracellular responses once extracellular stimuli are processed. One of the more critical is the extracellular signal-regulated kinases (ERK) pathway which plays a main role in neuronal changes, being implicated, i.e., in reward after cocaine consumption [15]. Also, cAMP response element binding protein (CREB) is crucial being its activation through phosphorylation (pCREB). Previous studies from our laboratory have suggested an enhancement of pCREB during morphine withdrawal in the NTS [16]. Besides, CREB regulates TH phosphorylation, limiting enzyme for DA synthesis.

2. Brain stress system and addiction

Brain stress system is composed of two different linked structures: hypothalamic-pituitary-adrenal (HPA) axis and the extended amygdala [17]. Both structures are activated during drug intake and during withdrawal, resulting in CRF and glucocorticoid release [18].

2.1 HPA axis

Also known as hypothalamic brain stress system, as its name suggests, it is divided in three components: the PVN, the pituitary, and the suprarenal glands [1, 12, 19]. In the PVN, CRF is released from the medial parvocellular subdivision to the median eminence reaching the pituitary (**Figure 1**) where it stimulates the synthesis and release of adrenocorticotropic hormone (ACTH) through CRF1R and CRF2R activation [20, 21]. Consequently, ACTH stimulates the synthesis and release of glucocorticoids from the adrenal glands. These glucocorticoids regulate the HPA axis through a negative feedback system once they interact with glucocorticoid (GR) and mineralocorticoid receptors (MR). Changes in this system are proposed to mediate transition from acute consumption to chronic consumption in

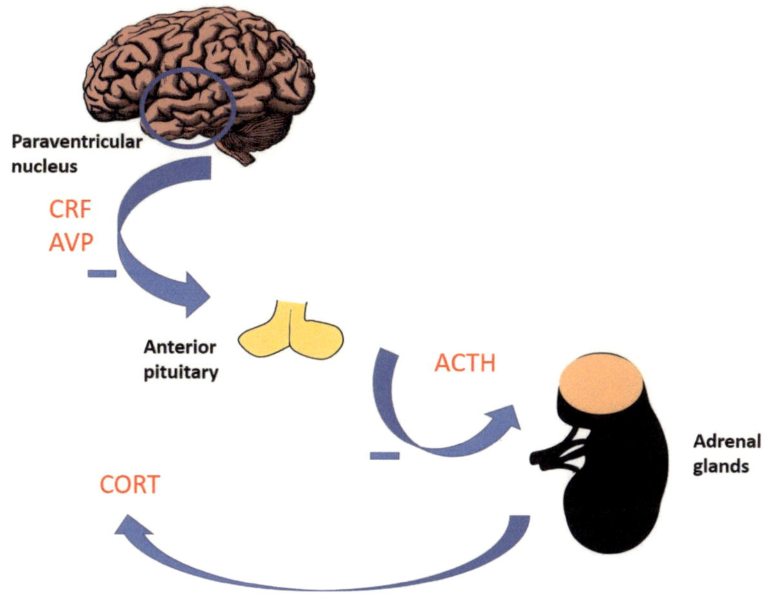

Figure 1.
Representation of the HPA axis. The hypothalamic brain stress system or HPA axis is composed by the PVN, the pituitary, and the suprarenal glands. CRF binds to CRF1R and CRF2R resulting in the activation of the pituitary which consequently, through ACTH, produces release of glucocorticoids (corticosterone, CORT) by the adrenal glands resulting in negative feedback over the previous steps.

addicted [12, 22]. Previous research has shown that different antagonists can block the negative state that come across during morphine withdrawal [23]. Besides, chronic exposure to opiates results in physic dependence and tolerance, and it is accompanied by enhanced ACTH and corticosterone release during morphine withdrawal [24]. Stressful situations can result in relapse in dependent or abstinent humans [25] and cause reinstatement of drug-seeking in different animal relapsing models [26].

2.2 Extended amygdala

The extrahypothalamic brain stress system or the extended amygdala (**Figure 2**) is composed of different nuclei as bed nucleus of the stria terminalis (BNST), central nucleus of the amygdala (CeA), and the shell of the NAc [27, 28]. These nuclei have similar functions and are responsible of connecting the limbic structures as hippocampus, basolateral amygdala, or the midbrain [12, 29]. Also, limbic structures mediate responses and behavior guiding the individuals according to memories [30]. Here, CRF receptors and CRF neuron cell bodies have been seen in BNST and CeA innervating each other and others as the NAc [28, 31, 32]. Therefore, CRF has a prominent role in this structure. Moreover, the extended amygdala is a key component in the acquisition and development of different negative symptoms through the release of CRF together with other neurotransmitters or peptides like NA or dynorphin [17, 33, 34]. In addition, extended amygdala is linked to the NTS (a noradrenergic nucleus) through innervations from there to the BNST, CeA, or the NAc [35, 36]. Thereupon, the extended amygdala, a part of the brain stress system, connects with the noradrenergic system and the dopaminergic pathways [37]. In fact, it has been suggested that activation of the brain stress system would result in sensibilization of the dopaminergic pathways [38, 39].

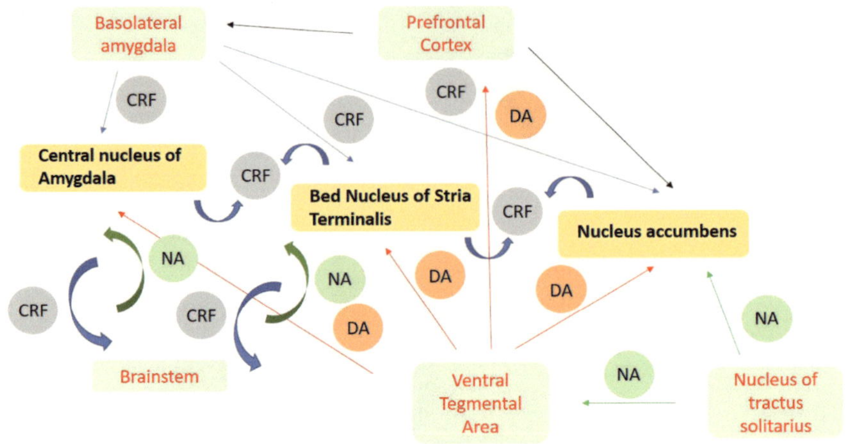

Figure 2.
Representation of the extended amygdala. The extrahypothalamic brain stress system or extended amygdala is shown here in a scheme with its main nuclei: BNST, CeA, and NAc. Noradrenergic innervations establish a feedforward loop between CRF and NA, which remains crucial for the development of drug addiction and relapses. Besides, there is dopaminergic innervation from ventral tegmental area to different nuclei establishing a relationship between NA system, DA system, and the brain stress system (hypothalamic and extrahypothalamic).

3. Role of glucocorticoids in addiction

Glucocorticoids are the final step of HPA axis, and their release takes place in response to stressful situations, becoming this activation one of the main mechanisms of adaption to stress [40]. Glucocorticoids make their function by interacting with two classes of receptors: MR or type I and GR or type II [41].

Whereas MR are located in limbic areas of the brain such as amygdala and also in the PVN or the locus coeruleus (LC) [42], GR have a more heterogeneous localization, with deep presence in the PVN, amygdala, or the hippocampus. MR have higher affinity for corticosterone than GR, but GR are activated when there are stressful facts differently to MR, which are important at basal levels. Both receptors have presence in the NTS, making this nucleus to be important in glucocorticoid effects [43]. Previous research has shown that MR blockade decreases self-administration of cocaine, suggesting a role for these receptors in addiction [44].

Moreover, stress affects GR, which are located through the dopaminergic pathways enhancing HPA axis and dopaminergic activity. In fact, glucocorticoids have been suggested to interact with a GRE site located in TH, resulting in the upregulation of TH synthesis and, finally, increasing DA release in the NAc [45]. Therefore, individuals with higher HPA axis activity would be more vulnerable to develop drug addiction [5].

4. Involvement of GR and MR in TH activity and phosphorylation in the NTS

The regulation in the biosynthesis of catecholamines by TH depends on its phosphorylation at serine 31 and serine 40. This has been proposed to be triggered by stressful situations considering that increased release of glucocorticoids results in uprising TH activity [46]. Moreover, morphine withdrawal induced by naloxone injection increased TH mRNA expression in the NTS and TH activity in the PVN [47]. Therefore, it was critical to elucidate if blocking GR and MR with mifepristone and spironolactone would affect TH phosphorylation during morphine withdrawal in the NTS. Results from our laboratory showed that TH phosphorylation at serine 31 and serine 40 was increased during naloxone-induced morphine withdrawal in rats, a fact that, together with the existence of enhanced NA turnover in the NTS during morphine withdrawal, suggests that TH regulates noradrenergic activity [24, 31, 48–50]. Besides, the blockade of GR with mifepristone, selective antagonist of GR, significantly attenuated the phosphorylation at serine 31, but not at serine 40 in the NTS during morphine withdrawal [48, 50], different to the results after blockade of MR with spironolactone. Pretreatment with this antagonist decreased phosphorylation of serine 31 in the NTS but not significantly [49, 50] (**Figure 3**). These results would suggest that enhanced glucocorticoid release during morphine withdrawal results in TH phosphorylation at serine 31, consequently, also in enhanced TH activity, and finally in higher catecholamine levels in the PVN, innervated by noradrenergic system.

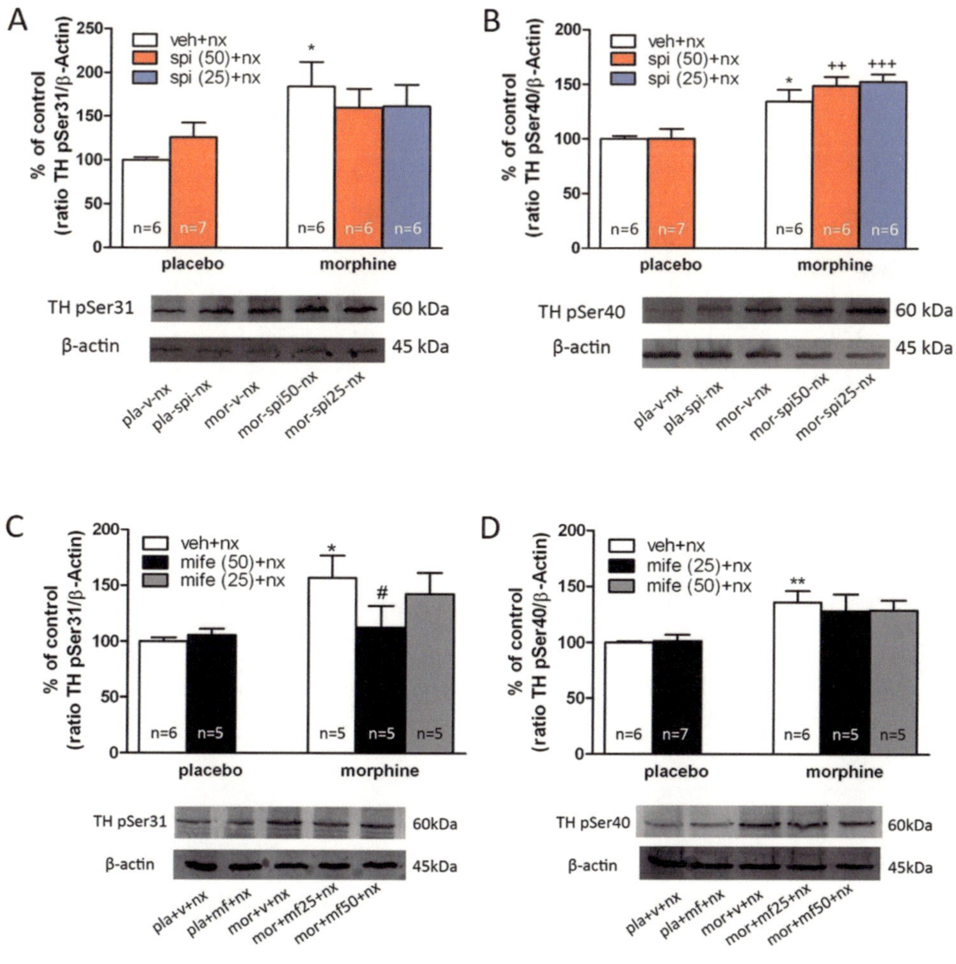

Figure 3.
Antagonization of TH phosphorylation at serine 31 by mifepristone (GR antagonist). Mifepristone (C) but not spironolactone (A) antagonized naloxone-induced morphine-withdrawal phosphorylation of TH at serine 31 in the NTS. Representative immunoblots of THpSer31 (A, C) and THpSer40 (B, D) in the NTS tissues isolated from placebo and morphine-dependent rats 60 min after administration of naloxone and the respective antagonist [mifepristone (C, D) or spironolactone (A, B)] or saline. Data represent the optical density of immunoreactive bands expressed as a percentage (%) of the mean ± SEM of placebo control band $^{*}P < 0.05$ *versus placebo + vehicle + naloxone;* $^{**}P < 0.01$ *versus placebo + vehicle + naloxone;* $^{\#}P < 0.05$ *versus morphine + vehicle + naloxone;* $^{++}P < 0.01$ *versus placebo + spironolactone+ naloxone;* $^{+++}P < 0.001$ *versus placebo + spironolactone + naloxone.*

5. Role of GR and MR in the activation of ERK pathway and CREB (via phosphorylation) in the NTS

Different studies have proposed the importance of ERK pathway in drug addiction, particularly, during morphine withdrawal [51, 52]. Protein Kinase C (PKC) regulates this pathway activated by the phosphorylation of ERKs [50, 52]. It is important to highlight that previous research has shown that ERK has a main role in the phosphorylation of TH at serine 31 in the NTS [53], supporting a synergic cooperation between the brain stress system, the noradrenergic system, and this pathway. GR but not MR blockade significantly decreased the enhanced activity (via phosphorylation) seen in pERK1 and pERK2 during morphine withdrawal in rats, supporting a role for glucocorticoids in activation of ERK pathway (**Figure 4**).

On the other hand, it is known that CREB has a main role in addiction to drugs of abuse as a transcription factor [54]. Nevertheless, CREB is the final step of protein kinase A (PKA) signaling pathway, although PKC pathway has been also proposed to be mediating its activation in the NTS [16]. As it happens with ERK,

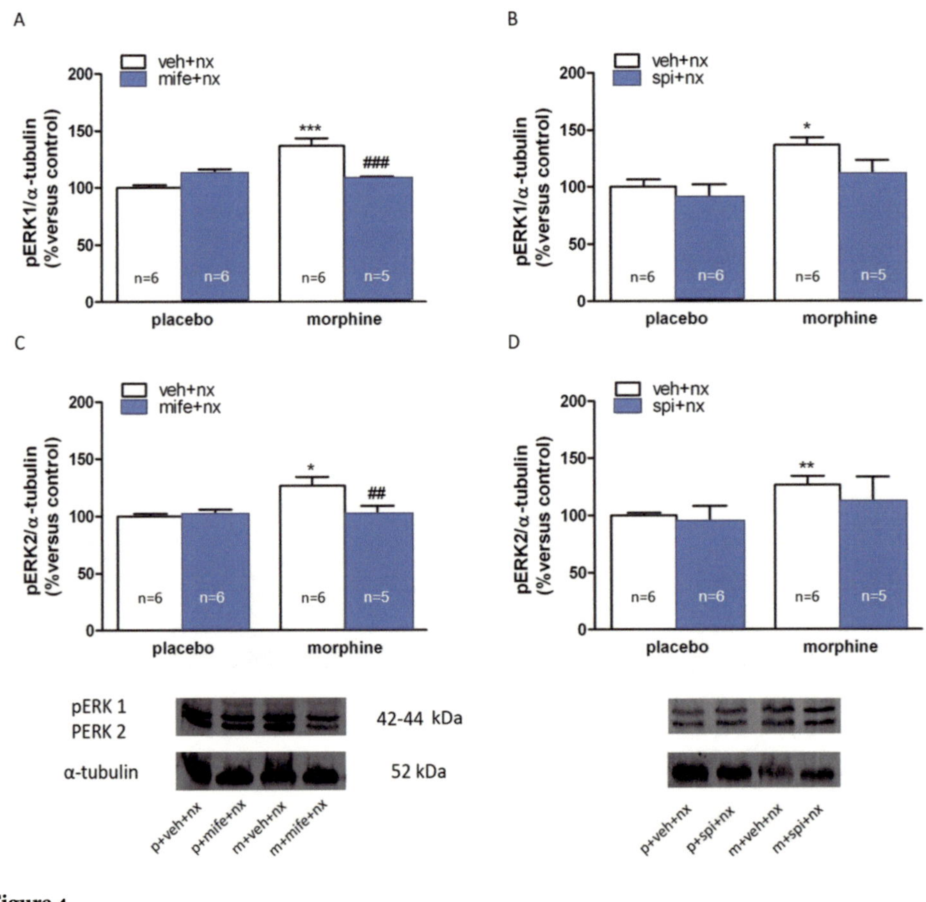

Figure 4.
Antagonization of ERK 1 and ERK 2 phosphorylation by mifepristone (GR antagonist). Mifepristone (A, C) but not spironolactone (B, D) antagonized naloxone-induced morphine-withdrawal phosphorylation of ERK 1 and ERK 2 in the NTS. Representative immunoblots of ERK 1 (A, B) and ERK 2 (C, D) in the NTS tissues isolated from placebo and morphine-dependent rats 60 min after administration of naloxone and the respective antagonist [mifepristone (A, C) or spironolactone (B, D)] or saline. Data represent the optical density of immunoreactive bands expressed as a percentage (%) of the mean ± SEM of placebo control band. $^{*}P < 0.05$ *versus placebo + vehicle+ naloxone;* $^{**}P < 0.01$ *versus placebo + vehicle + naloxone;* $^{*}P < 0.05$ *versus placebo + vehicle + naloxone* $^{\#\#}P < 0.01$ *versus morphine + vehicle + naloxone;* $^{\#\#\#}P < 0.001$ *versus morphine + vehicle + naloxone.*

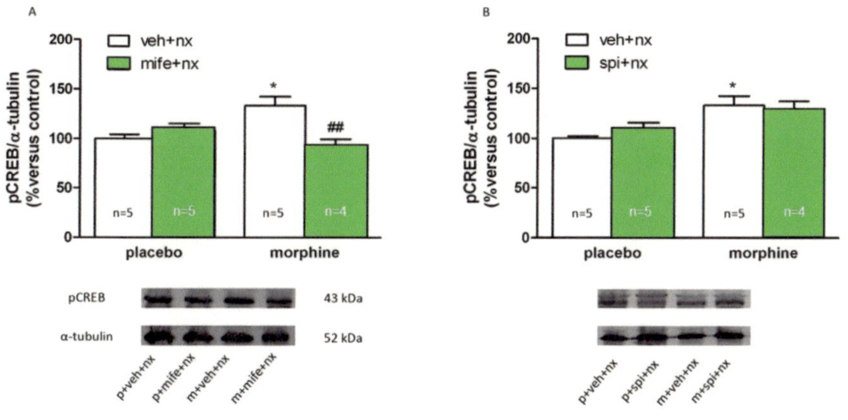

Figure 5.
*Antagonization of CREB phosphorylation by mifepristone (GR antagonist). Mifepristone (A) but not spironolactone (B) antagonized naloxone-induced morphine-withdrawal phosphorylation of CREB in the NTS. Representative immunoblots of pCREB in the NTS tissues isolated from placebo and morphine-dependent rats 60 min after administration of naloxone and the respective antagonist mifepristone (A) or spironolactone (B) or saline. Data represent the optical density of immunoreactive bands expressed as a percentage (%) of the mean ± SEM of placebo control band. *P < 0.05 versus placebo + vehicle + naloxone; ##P < 0.01 versus morphine + vehicle + naloxone.*

CREB is activated via phosphorylation, and it has been shown to be enhanced in the NTS during morphine withdrawal [16, 50]. Once again, GR but not MR blockade significantly decreased the phosphorylation of CREB seen during morphine withdrawal [50] (**Figure 5**). Therefore, GR would be implicated in CREB activation during morphine withdrawal in the NTS.

6. Conclusion

Previous research has shown that CRE (binding site for CREB) and GRE (binding site for GR) are present in the gene promoters that regulate activity of TH [55], setting a relationship between NA system, the HPA axis and the extended amygdala, and finally, CREB. In contrast, little was known about the mechanisms underlying this regulation. This review suggests that stressful situations as naloxone-induced morphine withdrawal would result in glucocorticoid release which would activate GR. Immediately, GR would produce an activation of PKC signaling pathway that would regulate ERK pathway and CREB activation (via phosphorylation) in the NTS. Finally, TH activity would be enhanced in the NTS through the activation of different sites as CRE or GRE resulting in catecholamine release in the PVN, supporting a main role for glucocorticoids and the GR in drug addiction.

Acknowledgements

This research was supported by a grant from the Ministerio de Economía, Industria y Competitividad (SAF2017-85679-R) and a grant from Fundación Séneca-Agencia de Ciencia y Tecnología de la Región de Murcia (20847/PI/18).

Conflict of interest

The authors declare no conflict of interest.

Author details

Javier Navarro-Zaragoza*, María Victoria Milanés and María Luisa Laorden
Faculty of Medicine, Department of Pharmacology, University of Murcia, Spain

*Address all correspondence to: jnavarrozaragoza@um.es

References

[1] Koob GF, Schulkin J. Addiction and stress: An allostatic view. Neuroscience and Biobehavioral Reviews. 2019;**106**: 245-262

[2] Koob GF, Volkow ND. Neurocircuitry of addiction. Neuropsychopharmacology. 2010;**35**:217-238

[3] Robinson TE, Berridge KC. Addiction. Annual Review of Psychology. 2003;**54**: 25-53

[4] Koob G, Kreek MJ. Stress, dysregulation of drug reward pathways, and the transition to drug dependence. The American Journal of Psychiatry. 2007;**164**:1149-1159

[5] Uhart M, Wand GS. Stress, alcohol and drug interaction: An update of human research. Addiction Biology. 2009;**14**:43-64

[6] Kalivas PW, O'Brien C. Drug addiction as a pathology of staged neuroplasticity. Neuropsychopharmacology. 2008;**33**:166-180

[7] Di Chiara G, Bassareo V. Reward system and addiction: What dopamine does and doesn't do. Current Opinion in Pharmacology. 2007;**7**:69-76

[8] Wise RA. Neurobiology of addiction. Current Opinion in Neurobiology. 1996;**6**:243-251

[9] Robbins TW, Everitt BJ. Neurobehavioural mechanisms of reward and motivation. Current Opinion in Neurobiology. 1996;**6**:228-236

[10] Hyman SE, Malenka RC. Addiction and the brain: The neurobiology of compulsion and its persistence. Nature Reviews. Neuroscience. 2001;**2**:695-703

[11] Koob GF, Simon EJ. The neurobiology of addiction: Where we have been and where we are going. Journal of Drug Issues. 2009;**39**:115-132

[12] Koob GF. Brain stress systems in the amygdala and addiction. Brain Research. 2009;**1293**:61-75

[13] Delfs JM, Zhu Y, Druhan JP, Aston-Jones G. Noradrenaline in the ventral forebrain is critical for opiate withdrawal-induced aversion. Nature. 2000;**403**:430-434

[14] Koob GF. Stress, corticotropin-releasing factor, and drug addiction. Annals of the New York Academy of Sciences. 1999;**897**:27-45

[15] Lu L, Hope BT, Dempsey J, Liu SY, Bossert JM, Shaham Y. Central amygdala ERK signalling pathway is critical to incubation of cocaine craving. Nature Neuroscience. 2005;**8**:212-219

[16] Martín F, Laorden ML, Milanes MV. Morphine withdrawal regulates phosphorylation of cAMP response element binding protein (CREB) through PKC in the nucleus tractus solitarius-A2 catecholaminergic neurons. Journal of Neurochemistry. 2009;**110**:1422-1432

[17] Goodman A. Neurobiology of addiction. An integrated review. Biochemical Pharmacology. 2008;**75**:266-322

[18] Koob GF, Le Moal M. Neurobiological mechanisms for opponent motivational processes in addiction. Philosophical Transactions of the Royal Society B: Biological Sciences. 2008;**363**:3113-3123

[19] Smith SM, Vale WW. The role of the hypothalamic-pituitary-adrenal axis in neuroendocrine responses to stress. Dialogues in Clinical Neuroscience. 2006;**8**:383-395

[20] Lowery EG, Spanos M, Navarro M, Lyons AM, Hodge CW, Thiele TE. CRF-1 antagonist and CRF-2 agonist decrease binge-like ethanol drinking in C57BL/6J mice independent of the

HPA axis. Neuropsychopharmacology. 2010;**35**:1241-1252

[21] Lowery EG, Thiele TE. Pre-clinical evidence that corticotropin-releasing factor (CRF) receptor antagonists are promising targets for pharmacological treatment of alcoholism. CNS and Neurological Disorders Drug Targets. 2010;**9**:77-86

[22] Shalev U, Erb S, Shaham Y. Role of CRF and other neuropeptides in stress-induced reinstatement of drug seeking. Brain Research. 2010;**1314**:15-28

[23] Koob GF. The dark of emotion: The addiction perspective. European Journal of Pharmacology. 2015;**753**:73-87

[24] Navarro-Zaragoza J, Núñez C, Ruiz-Medina J, Laorden ML, Valverde O, Milanés MV. CRF(2) mediates the increased noradrenergic activity in the hypothalamic paraventricular nucleus and the negative state of morphine withdrawal in rats. British Journal of Pharmacology. 2011;**162**:851-862

[25] Sinha R. How does stress increase risk of drug abuse and relapse? Psychopharmacology. 2001;**158**:343-359

[26] Erb S, Shaham Y, Stewart J. Stress reinstates cocaine seeking behaviour after prolonged extinction and a drug-free period. Psychopharmacology. 1996;**128**:408-412

[27] Volkow ND, Michaelides M, Baler R. The neuroscience of drug reward and addiction. Physiological Reviews. 2019;**99**:2115-2140

[28] Koob GF, Le Moal M. Addiction and the brain antireward system. Annual Review of Physiology. 2008;**59**:29-53

[29] Edwards S, Koob GF. Experimental psychiatric illness and drug abuse models: From human to animal, an overview. Methods in Molecular Biology. 2012;**829**:31-48

[30] Daviu N, Bruchas MR, Moghaddam B, Sandi C, Beyeler A. Neurobiological links between stress and anxiety. Neurobiol Stress. 2019;**11**:100191

[31] Navarro-Zaragoza J, Núñez C, Laorden ML, Milanes MV. Effects of corticotropin-releasing factor receptor-1 (CRF1R) antagonists on the brain stress system responses to morphine withdrawal. Molecular Pharmacology. 2010;**77**:864-873

[32] Jiang Z, Shivakumar R, Justice NJ. CRF signaling between neurons in the paraventricular nucleus of the hypothalamus (PVN) coordinates stress responses. Neurobiol Stress. 2019;**11**:100192

[33] Bale TL, Vale WW. CRF and CRF receptors: Role in stress responsivity and other behaviors. Annual Review of Pharmacology and Toxicology. 2004;**44**:525-557

[34] Orozco-Cabal L, Pollandt S, Liu J, Shinnick-Gallagher P, Gallagher JP. Regulation of synaptic transmission by CRF receptors. Reviews in the Neurosciences. 2006;**17**:279-307

[35] Lavicky J, Dunn AJ. Corticotropin-releasing factor stimulates catecholamine release in hypothalamus and prefrontal cortex in freely moving rats as assessed by microdialysis. Journal of Neurochemistry. 1993;**60**:602-612

[36] Martin F, Nunez C, Marin MT, Laorden ML, Kovacs KJ, Milanes MV. Involvement of noradrenergic transmission in the PVN on CREB activation, TORC1 levels, and pituitary-adrenal Axis activity during morphine withdrawal. PLoS One. 2012;**7**:e31119, 57

[37] Delfs JM, Zhu Y, Druhan JP, Aston-Jones GS. Origin of noradrenergic afferents to the shell subregion of the nucleus accumbens: Anterograde and retrograde tract-tracing studies in the rat. Brain Research. 1998;**806**:127-140

[38] de Jong IME, Steenbergen PJ, de Kloet ER. Behavioral sensitization to cocaine: Cooperation between glucocorticoids and epinephrine. Psychopharmacology. 2009;**204**:693-703

[39] Barrot M, Abrous DN, Marinelli M, Rouge-Pont F, Le Moal M, Piazza PV. Influence of glucocorticoids on dopaminergic transmission in the rat dorsolateral striatum. The European Journal of Neuroscience. 2001;**13**:812-818

[40] Tronche F, Kellendonk C, Kretz O, Gass P, Anlag K, Orban PC, et al. Disruption of the glucocorticoid receptor gene in the nervous system results in reduced anxiety. Nature Genetics. 1999;**23**:99-103

[41] Noguchi T, Makino S, Matsumoto R, Nakayama S, Nishiyama M, Terada Y, et al. Regulation of Glucocorticoid Receptor transcription and nuclear translocation during single and repeated immobilization stress. Endocrinology. 2010;**151**:4344-4355

[42] Marinelli PW, Harding S, Funk D, Juzytsch W, Le AD. The influence of stress on the alcohol deprivation effect and of stress-associated cues on reinstatement in the rat. Alcoholism, Clinical and Experimental Research. 2006;**30**:27

[43] Joels M, Baram TZ. The neuro-symphony of stress. Nature Reviews. Neuroscience. 2009;**10**:459-484

[44] Fiancette JF, Balado E, Piazza PV, Deroche-Gamonet V. Mifepristone and spironolactone differently alter cocaine intravenous self-administration and cocaine-induced locomotion in C57BL/6J mice. Addiction Biology. 2010;**15**:81-87

[45] Piazza PV, Le Moal M. Glucocorticoids as a biological substrate of reward: Physiological and pathophysiological implications. Brain Research Reviews. 1997;**25**:359-372

[46] Hagerty T, Fernandez E, Lynch K, Wang SS, Morgan WW, Strong R. Interaction of a glucocorticoid-responsive element with regulatory sequences in the promoter region of the mouse tyrosine hydroxylase gene. Journal of Neurochemistry. 2001;**78**:1379-1388

[47] Benavides M, Laorden ML, García-Borrón JC, Milanés MV. Regulation of tyrosine hydroxilase levels and activity and Fos expression during opioid withdrawal in the hypothalamic PVN and medulla oblongata catecholaminergic cell groups innervating the PVN. The European Journal of Neuroscience. 2003;**17**:103-112

[48] Navarro-Zaragoza J, Hidalgo JM, Laorden ML, Milanés MV. Glucocorticoids participate in the opiate-withdrawal-induced stimulation of rats NTS noradrenergic activity and in the somatic signs of morphine withdrawal. British Journal of Pharmacology. 2012;**166**:2136-2147

[49] Navarro-Zaragoza J, Laorden ML, Milanés MV. Spironolactone decreases the somatic signs of opiate withdrawal by blocking the mineralocorticoid receptors (MR). Toxicology. 2014;**326**:36-43

[50] Navarro-Zaragoza J, Laorden ML, Milanés MV. Glucocorticoid receptor but not mineralocorticoid receptor mediates the activation of ERK pathway and CREB during morphine withdrawal. Addiction Biology. 2017;**22**:342-353

[51] Cao JL, He JH, Ding HL, Zeng YM. Activation of the spinal ERK signalling pathways contributes naloxone-precipitated withdrawal in morphine dependents rats. Pain. 2005;**118**:336-349

[52] Almela P, Milanés MV, Laorden ML. Activation of the ERK signalling pathway contributes to the adaptive changes in rat hearts during naloxone-induced morphine withdrawal.

British Journal of Pharmacology. 2007;**151**:787-797

[53] Dunkley PR, Bobrovskaya L, Graham ME, von Nagy-Felsobuki E, Dickson PW. Tyrosine hydroxylase phosphorylation: Regulation and consequences. Journal of Neurochemistry. 2004;**91**:1025-1043

[54] Nestler EJ. Celullar basis of memory for addiction. Dialogues in Clinical Neuroscience. 2013;**15**(4):431-443

[55] Rani CSS, Elango N, Wang S, Kobayashi K, Strong R. Identification of an activator protein-1-like sequence as the glucocorticoid response element in the rat tyrosine hydroxylase gene. Molecular Pharmacology. 2009;**75**:589-598

Chapter 5

Corticotrophin-Releasing Factor (CRF) through CRF1 Receptor Facilitates the Expression of Morphine-Related Positive and Aversive Memory in Mice

Pilar Almela, Juan A. García-Carmona,
Elena Martínez-Laorden, María V. Milanés
and María L. Laorden

Abstract

Different studies have elucidated the mechanisms underlying the formation and expression of drug-related cue memories; corticotrophin-releasing factor (CRF) plays a critical role in reward- and aversion-driven associative learning. In the present chapter, we have evaluated whether CP-154,526, a selective CRF1 receptor (CRF1R) antagonist, or genetic deletion of CRF1R (KO mice) have comparable effects on conditioned place preference (CPP) and conditioned place aversion (CPA) learning. We also investigated CP-154,526 effects on morphine-induced CPP activation of CRF, CREB phosphorylation, and thioredoxin (Trx1) expression in dentate gyrus (DG), a brain region involved in memory consolidation, and the role of hypothalamic-pituitary-adrenocortical (HPA) axis in CPA expression and extinction. The CRF1R antagonist abolished the acquisition of morphine CPP, Trx-1 and BDNF increased expression, and pCREB/Trx-1 co-localization in the DG. The increase in adrenocorticotropic hormone (ACTH) plasma levels observed after CPA expression was attenuated in CRF1R KO mice, suggesting a role of HPA axis in aversive memories. Altogether, these results suggest a critical role of CRF, through CRF1R, in molecular changes involved in memory formation and consolidation and may facilitate the development of effective treatments for opioid addiction.

Keywords: conditioned place preference, conditioned place aversion, morphine, hippocampus, CRF, HPA axis

1. Introduction

Drug addiction is a chronic brain disease with a high rate of relapse [1–3]. Despite years of abstinence from drugs, relapse can occur when addicts encounter cues, including people or places, associated with their prior drug use [4]. Drug-associated memory can persist throughout the lifetime of a patient; therefore, the elimination of this kind of memory is considered to be crucial for the treatment of drug addiction.

In organism and human models, drug reward can be assessed using a Pavlovian conditioning procedure known as conditioned place preference/conditioned place aversion (CPP/CPA) [5–7]. CPP for the drug-paired environment is predicted by self-reported measures of drug liking in humans [6]. CPA for the drug-paired environment is used to infer the dysphoric properties of drugs, including opioid receptor antagonists [8]. Many neurotransmitters, neurotrophic factors, and protein kinases have been delineated in the regulation of the formation and expression of drug-associated reward memories and withdrawal-associated aversive memories [9–13].

Corticotrophin-releasing factor (CRF) in the brain plays a critical role in reward- and aversion-driven associative learning. However, it is not clear whether it does this by a common mechanism or by separated mechanisms that can be dissociated. The knowledge of these mechanisms could lead to more effective treatments for addictive processes. CRF and its CRF1 receptor (CRF1R) are widely distributed and in a highly conserved way in several brain regions, including the hippocampal formation, involved in reward reinforcement, craving and aversive effects of drug of abuse [14–17]. At the extrahypothalamic level, CRF acts as a neuroregulator of the behavioral and emotional integration of environmental and endogenous stimuli associated with drug dependence [18, 19]. In the hippocampal dentate gyrus (DG), an important brain region involved in saving similar experiences and contexts [20], CRF is released from inhibitory interneurons [21] through CRF1R [14] by environmental signals. CRF1R activation stimulates Gαs protein, promoting the induction of the protein kinase A/cAMP response element binding protein (CREB) pathway [22]. CREB activity in the brain is critical for learning and memory processes [23], and it has been reported to be involved in the expression of opioid dependence. The activation of CREB, as one of the main downstream effectors of extracellular signal-regulated kinase (ERK), accelerates the transcription of CREB-dependent genes such as the brain-derived neurotrophic factor (BDNF). With respect to hypothalamus, CRF release from paraventricular nucleus (PVN) controls the hypothalamic-pituitary-adrenal (HPA) axis responses to stress and drug addiction [24–26]. CRF neurons in the PVN and CRF fibber in DG have direct connexion with dopaminergic neurons located in the ventral tegmental area (VTA) projecting to nucleus accumbens (NAc) [27, 28].

2. Role of CRF in the rewarding effects of morphine

CPP is an animal model widely used to evaluate the correlation between contexts and drugs. Different substances of abuse display differential ability to produce CPP. Opiates induce strong CPP over a wide range of experimental conditions [5]. Previous studies from our laboratory [29–32] and others [33, 34] have demonstrated that morphine administration evokes significant CPP for the drug-associated environment. Different neurobiological substrates have been involved in the rewarding properties of drugs of abuse, although the mesolimbic dopaminergic pathway has been pointed out to be the critical system for drug reward. Recently, it has been suggested that PVN may have a role in the reinforcing effects of opioids [35]. Various studies have elucidated the mechanisms underlying the formation and expression of drug-related cue memories. CRF in the brain plays a critical role in reward-driven associative learning. During the formation or consolidation process (CPP expression), the majority of the CRF-positive neurons in the PVN, central nucleus of amygdale (CeA), and bed nucleus of stria terminalis (BNST) coexpresses pCREB after morphine-induced CPP, suggesting that drug-paired context could trigger neuronal activity in the brain stress system [29]. Morphine-treated mice in their home cage do not show any changes in total CRF/CREB positive neurons, indicating that the exposure to drug-paired environments is necessary for CRF activation in the brain stress system [29]. Anatomical and functional studies reveal connections between CRF and the mesolimbic dopaminergic system. Thus, VTA and NAc receive CRF-positive projections from the PVN and stress extrahypothalamic areas [36, 37], which have been proposed to regulate dopamine release. The rewarding effect of morphine (CPP expression) is decreased by pretreatment with CP-154,526, a selective CRF1 antagonist, suggesting an important role of CRF/CRF1 receptor in memory formation and consolidation [30].

2.1 Implications of different signaling pathways in the rewarding effects of morphine. Role of CRF1 receptors

Hippocampus is a brain region known to participate in associative processes such as declarative memory, and PVN is an important stress area. Both structures are related with mesolimbic pathways [38]. Our group has studied the implication of different signaling pathways in both areas, because the understanding of how the formation of drug-reward memories alters the neurobiology of the hippocampal DG and PVN, and may shed light on the later and more persistent aspect of addiction.

The transcription factor CREB is critical in the conversion from short-term to long-term memory, and it is involved in the creation of long-term memory. Learning and memory and drug addiction share certain intracellular signaling pathways and depend on activation of CREB [39]. According to previous studies [40, 41], our laboratory has demonstrated that the number of pCREB positive neurons in PVN and DG is significantly increased after morphine-induced CPP expression (**Figure 1**). Since CRF1R is coupled to stimulatory G protein Gαs and can thus activate PKA and, subsequently, CREB [22], our group has investigated if CRF1R signaling is involved in CREB activity after morphine-induced CPP. Administration of the CRF1R antagonist, CP-154,526, completely revoked pCREB positive neuron enhancement induced by morphine in PVN and slightly in DG. CREB involvement in morphine dependence has been previously supported by studies demonstrating that CREB mutant mice do not respond to the reinforcing properties of morphine in a conditioned place preference paradigm [42], suggesting that specific CREB functions are necessary for the rewarding properties of this drug.

Although it is known that CRF signaling is involved in the drug withdrawal-induced anxiogenic-like and negative behavioral response [43], no definitive data are available about the role in the positive reinforcing properties of opiates. CRF-immunoreactive fibers densely innervate many intrahypothalamic and extrahypothalamic brain areas, such as hippocampus. Besides, CRF, through CRF1R, increases neuronal activity propagation from DG, the classical hippocampal input region, to the hypothalamic structure CA1 [44]. CRF is present in GABAergic hippocampal neurons of the pyramidal cells [14]. The supramammillary (SuM) region of the hypothalamus acts a connection nucleus between limbic and hypothalamic structures involved in controlling cognitive aspects [45]. Thus, SuM sends robust and direct inputs to DG. For example, it has been shown that mild stress could activate the SuM cells that project to the hippocampus [46]. Our group has previously shown that most of the CRF positive neurons in PVN coexpresses pCREB during morphine CPP. In addition, we have observed an enhancement in CRF fibers density in DG after morphine administration. Both changes were antagonized by injection of CP-154,526 (**Figure 2**). CRF binding to CRF1R results in activation of heterotrimeric G-proteins. The physiological functions of CRF1R in the central nervous system and in the periphery have been mainly associated to an increase in intracellular cAMP levels. This is consistent with a predominant coupling to Gαs

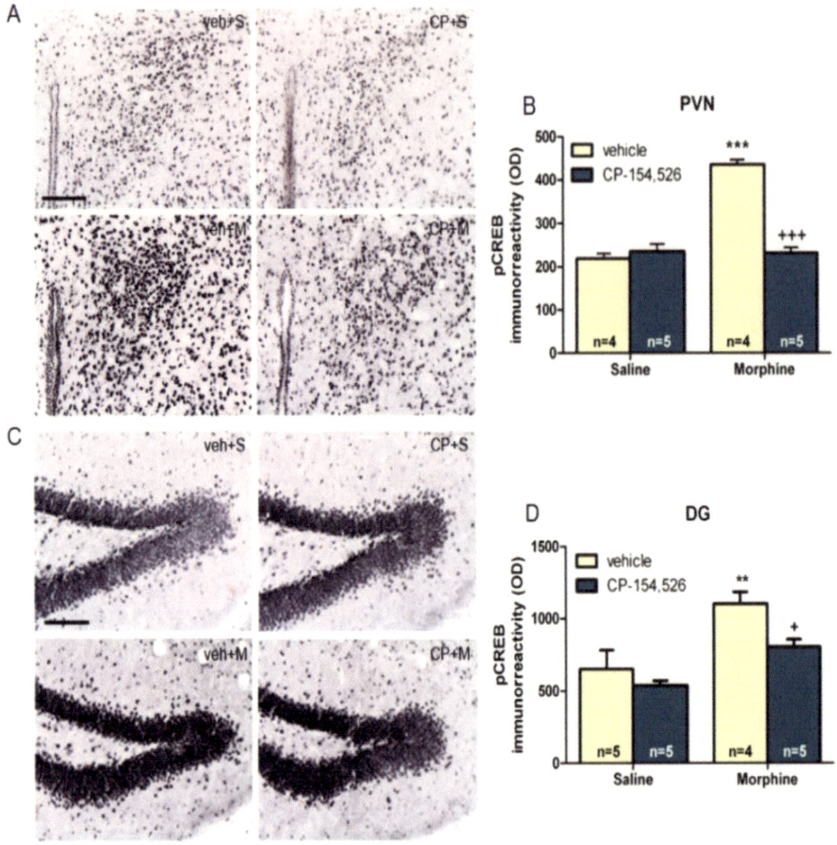

Figure 1.
*CREB activation in PVN (A) and DG (C) after morphine-induced CPP. Scale bar 100 μm. Quantitative analysis of pCREB immunodetection in PVN (B) and DG (D). Data are expressed as mean ± SEM. **$p < 0.01$, ***$p < 0.001$ versus vehicle (veh) + saline (S); +$p < 0.05$, +++$p < 0.001$ versus veh + morphine (M). CP-154,526 (CP). Optical density (OD).*

(cAMP/PKA/CREB). However, CRF through CRFR1 is capable of activating other Gα types such as Gαs and activate inositol triphosphate (IP3) cascade. An enhancement in the concentration of secondary messengers (cAMP, IP3, and Ca^{2+}) in cells, induced by CRF1R agonists, promotes the activation of several transcriptional factors such as CREB, AP-1, NF-κB, and the calcium response element (CARE) [47–53]. In this sense, the antagonist of the CRF1R, CP-154,526, by blocking the postsynaptic CRF1R, inhibited CREB phosphorylation in PVN and DG. Moreover, morphine treatment induced an increase in CRF fiber immunodetection in DG, suggesting an elevated CRF release, which was prevented by pretreatment with this antagonist. Since CRF1R activation increases Ca^{2+} levels, it is possible that CP-154,526 inhibits CRF release by blocking presynaptic CRF1R in PVN.

Several evidences suggest that CREB phosphorylation represents a site of convergence for various signaling pathways and alters gene expression [40]. CREB activation can also be regulated by the family of the redox protein Trx-1 [54]. In addition to its antioxidant activity, Trx-1 has been shown to play a crucial role in cellular signaling by controlling several important members of the signal transduction pathway. Thus, NF-κB, p38 mitogen-activated protein kinases, activator protein-1, CREB (as mentioned before), estrogen receptor, glucocorticoid receptor, and p53 are the targets of Trx-1 [55]. Data from our laboratory have shown that morphine-induced CPP increases Trx-1 expression in DG (**Figure 3**). Trx-1 might activate CREB

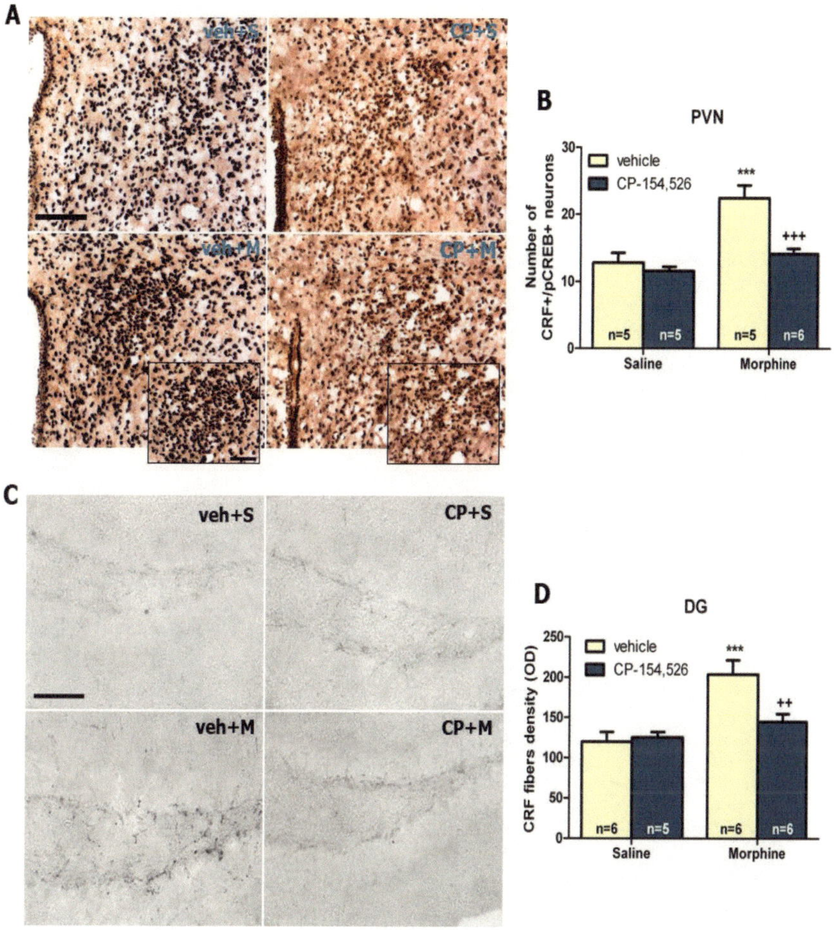

Figure 2.
*CRF/pCREB double-labeling photomicrographs in PVN (A). The upper right side of the figure shows the quantitative analysis of double-labeled neurons (B). CRF fiber photomicrographs in the DG (C). The down right side of the figure shows the CRF fiber density in the DG (D). Scale bar 100 or 50 μm. Data are expressed as mean ± SEM. ***p < 0.001 versus vehicle (veh) + saline (S); ++p < 0.01, +++p < 0.001 versus veh + morphine (M). CP-154,526 (CP). Optical density (OD).*

phosphorylation, thus increasing the rewarding effects of morphine. In agreement with our results, other studies have also observed an increased Trx-1 expression following morphine or methamphetamine administration [56]. Upregulation of CREB activity induced by methamphetamine was suppressed by Trx-1siRNA, which suggests that Trx-1 is necessary for CREB activation [55, 56]. Moreover, morphine-induced Trx-1 expression is blocked by naloxone, indicating that morphine induces Trx-1 expression via activating opioid receptors [57]. Results from our laboratory showing a positive relationship between morphine rewarding effects, and Trx-1 expression are in contrast with another study [58] demonstrating that geranylgeranylacetone induces Trx-1 and, concomitantly, reduces morphine-induced CPP. These variations could be explained by the differential regulating roles of NAc and hippocampus. Besides, CREB expression has been shown to be increased in hippocampus but decreased in NAc after morphine conditioning [40], which suggests that CREB activity is differently regulated depending on the brain area studied. Our investigations have demonstrated a large number of pCREB/Trx-1 double-labeled neurons in DG (**Figure 3**). These neuron colocalizations in DG suggest that CREB might be activated by Trx-1 in this brain nucleus involved in memory consolidation processes.

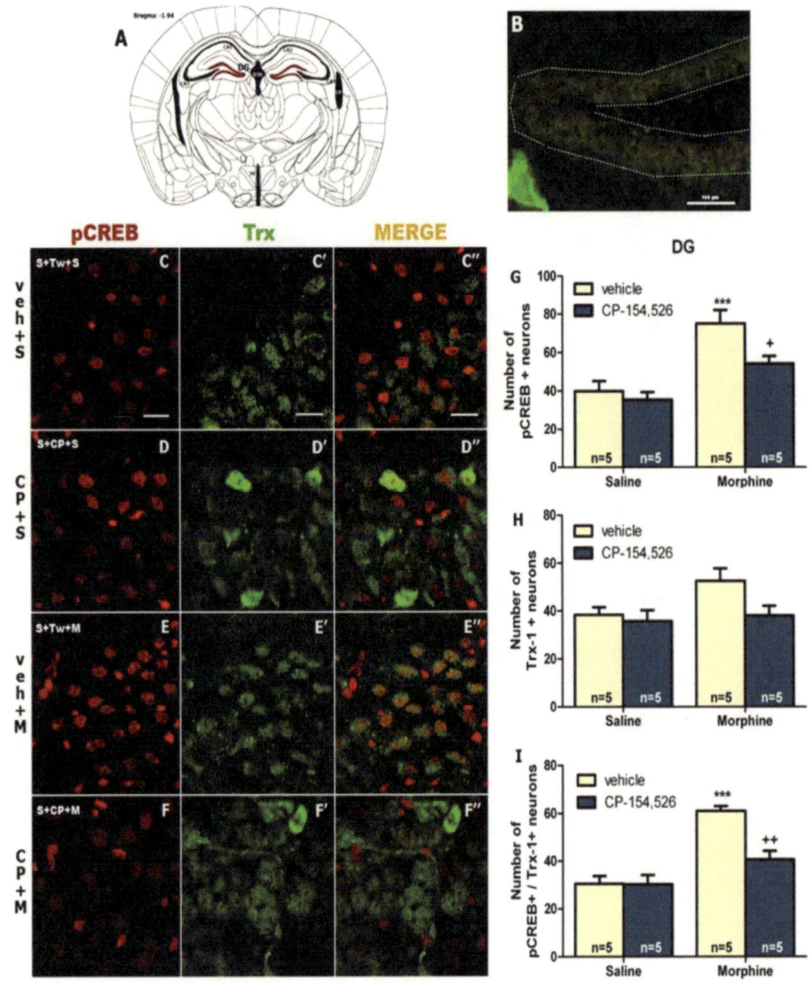

Figure 3.
*Characterization of pCREB and Trx-1 immunostaining in the dentate gyrus (DG) after morphine-induced CPP. (A) Schematic illustration showing the analyzed region of the DG (diagram modified from Franklin & Paxinos) [59]. Coordinate −1.94 mm from Bregma. (B) High-magnification image of a mouse midbrain coronal section immunostained for pCREB and Trx-1. Scale bar 100 μm. Representative confocal images of pCREB (red) (C–F) and Trx-1 (green) (C′–F′). Colocalization (pCREB/Trx-1) is shown in C″–F″ by yellow-orange neurons in the merged images. Scale bar 20 μm. Graphs on the right indicate the mean total number of pCREB (G), Trx-1 (H), and double-labeled (pCREB/Trx-1) neurons (I). Data are expressed as mean ± SEM. ***$p < 0.001$ versus vehicle (veh) + saline (S); +$p < 0.05$, ++$p < 0.01$ versus veh + morphine (M). CP-154,526 (CP).*

Due to the important role of TRX-1 in regulating the cellular redox balance, the induction of TRX-1 expression following morphine CPP could be associated to a mechanism of neural protection against a stressful situation.

Pretreatment with CP-154,526 completely blocks morphine-induced CPP elevation of Trx-1 expression in DG (**Figure 3**).

We have also shown an increase in the number of pCREB neurons coexpressing Trx-1 following morphine-induced CPP, so CRF1R could be involved in CREB phosphorylation, probably through a Trx-1-dependent way. The exact mechanism by which the CRF system participates in Trx-1 signaling regulation in DG is not completely understood. One possible explanation could indicate that pCREB binds to CRE in the 5′-upstream sequence of Trx-1 gene, thus inducing Trx-1 expression to regulate its phosphorylation. In agreement with this hypothesis, other authors have demonstrated that ephedrine promotes Trx-1 expression via the β-adrenergic receptor/cyclic AMP/PKA/DARPP-32 signaling pathway [60]. Besides, methamphetamine-induced CREB activity in rat pheochromocytoma cells was shown to be regulated by Trx-1 [56].

As shown in **Figure 4**, morphine-induced CPP increases the number of pCREB-positive neurons in PVN, an increase that was blocked by CP-154,526 treatment. However, there are no changes in the number of Trx-1 positive neurons or in the double labeled neurons (pCREB/Trx-1).

On the other hand, BDNF, an important neurotrophin for synaptic plasticity, is one of the molecular candidates underlying the development of persistent

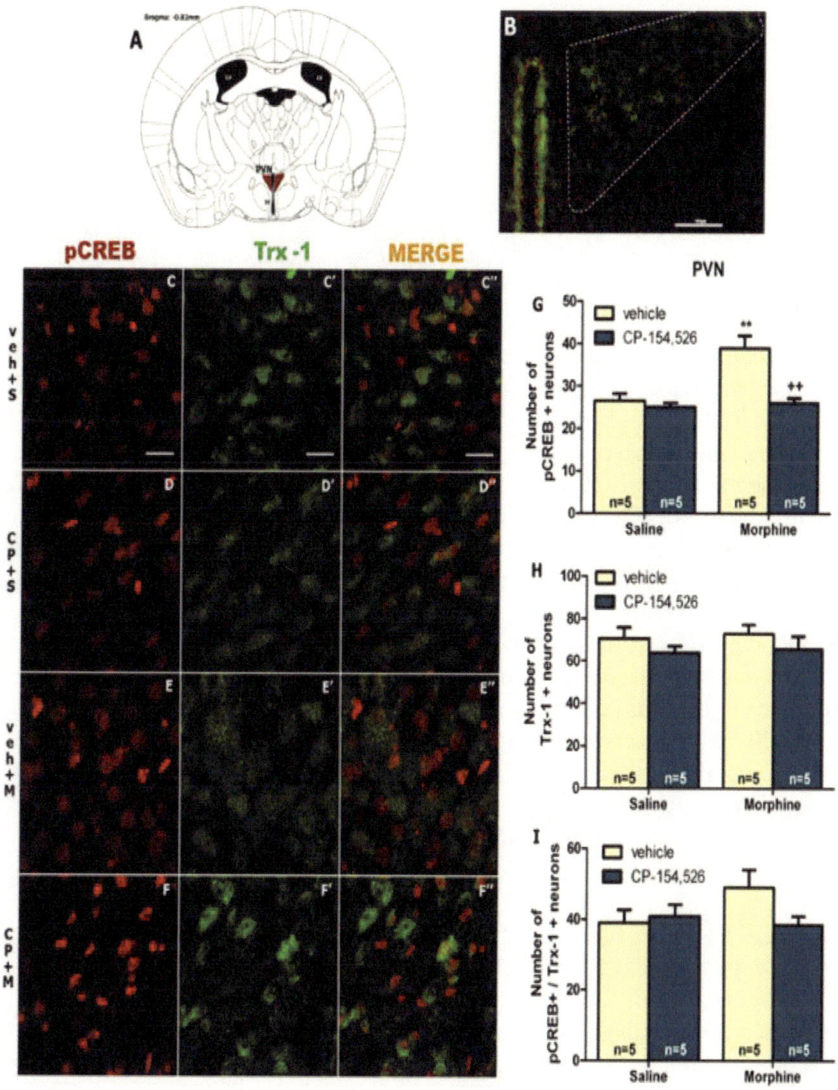

Figure 4.
*Characterization of pCREB and Trx-1 immunostaining in the paraventricular nucleus (PVN) after morphine-induced CPP. (A) Schematic illustration showing the analyzed region of the PVN (diagram modified from Franklin & Paxinos) [59]. Coordinate −0.82 mm from Bregma. (B) High-magnification image of a mouse midbrain coronal section immunostained for pCREB and Trx-1. Scale bar 100 μm. Representative confocal images of pCREB (red) (C–F) and Trx-1 (green) (C′–F′). Colocalization (pCREB/Trx-1) is shown in C″–F″ by yellow-orange neurons in the merged images. Scale bar 20 μm. Graphs on the right indicate the mean total number of pCREB (G), Trx-1 (H), and double-labeled (pCREB/Trx-1) neurons (I). Data are expressed as mean ± SEM. **$p < 0.01$, versus vehicle (veh) + saline (S); ++$p < 0.01$, versus veh + morphine (M). CP-154,526 (CP).*

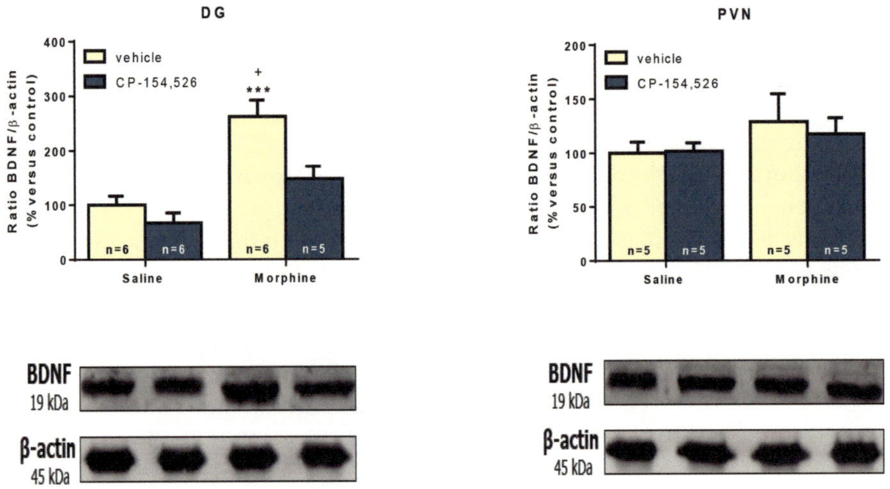

Figure 5.
*Western-blotting analysis of BDNF in the dentate gyrus (DG) and paraventricular nucleus (PVN) from animals pretreated with vehicle (veh) or CP-154,526 (CP) before saline or morphine. The immunoreactivity corresponding to BDNF is expressed as a percentage of that in the control group defined as 100% value. ***$p < 0.001$ versus morphine + CP; $+p < 0.05$ versus saline + veh.*

neuroplastic adaptation that regulates drug addiction [61]. Several lines of evidence indicate that chronic morphine treatment triggers ERK activation in different brain regions [62]. ERK phosphorylates CREB and active (phosphorylated) CREB stimulates the expression of target genes, including BDNF [63–65]. Chronic morphine use has been shown to increase the expression of BDNF in the NAc and hippocampus [61, 66, 67]. According to these data, our findings demonstrated that morphine-induced CPP activates BDNF signaling in the DG without any changes in the saline group (**Figure 5**), demonstrating that repeated morphine with context exposure, but not merely the context, increases BDNF expression in DG, suggesting that BDNF is implicated in drug-induced contextual memory formation. Therefore, BDNF is a crucial signal molecule involved in morphine dependence. However, whether this molecule is regulated in a CRF1R-dependent manner remains largely unknown: CP-154,526 attenuated CREB-BDNF expression (**Figures 4** and **5**) and prevented morphine-induced CPP [29]. Taken together, CRF1R-mediated CREB-BDNF signaling changes may regulate morphine reward through modulating contextual memory in the hippocampus.

3. Role of CRF1 receptor in the aversive effects induced by naloxone-precipitated withdrawal

The physical component of morphine withdrawal syndrome can be assessed by scoring some somatic withdrawal signs after morphine exposure [68]. Recent results from our group have demonstrated significant alterations in some morphine withdrawal signs such as body weight loss, rearing, rubbing, grooming, diarrhea, freezing, and time to first immobility in wild type morphine-withdrawn animals compared with controls treated with saline (**Figure 6**). Besides, and in agreement with previous studies [69–71], our laboratory has shown that body weight loss (**Figure 6H**), freezing (**Figure 6F**), and diarrhea (**Figure 6E**) are significantly attenuated in CRF1R KO mice although an increase in jumping in CRF1R KO mice was observed (**Figure 6A**), as it has been described previously by other authors [72]. Jumping is a sensitive and commonly used index of naloxone-induced withdrawal [73–76]. However, it is

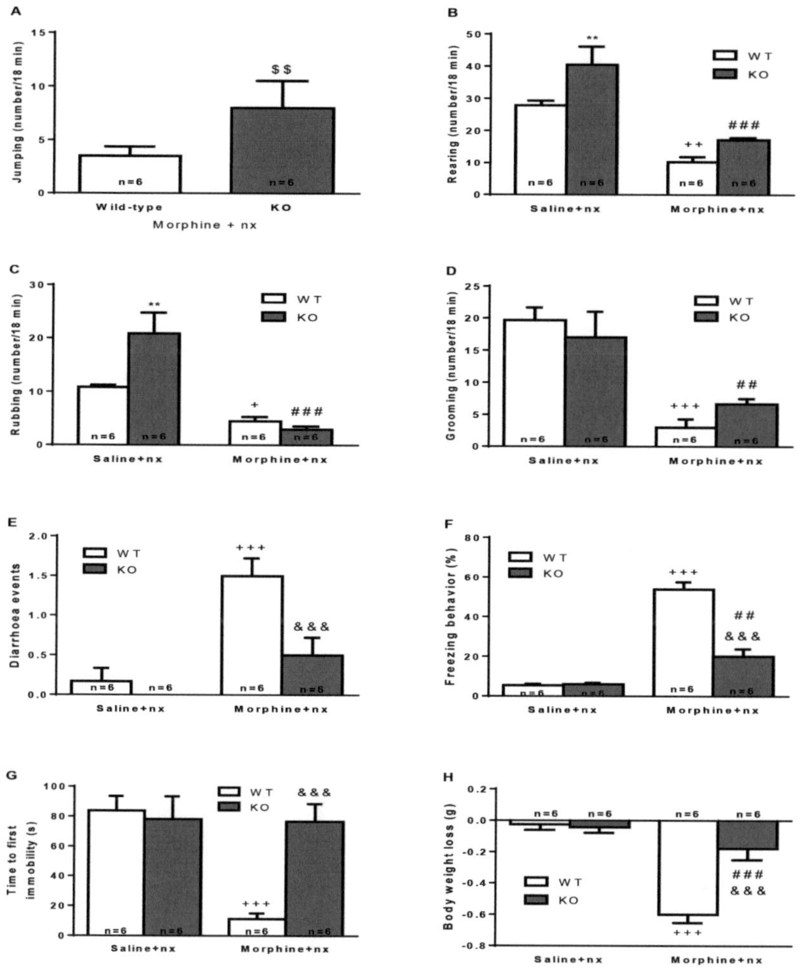

Figure 6.
*Behavior effects by naloxone (nx)-precipitated morphine withdrawal in wild type (WT) or knockout (CRF1R KO) mice. The following somatic signs, (A) jumping, (B) rearing, (C) rubbing, (D) grooming, (E) diarrhea, (F) freezing behavior, and (H) body weight loss, induced after nx (1 mg/kg, s.c.)-injection to morphine or saline-treated mice during 18 min, were evaluated. The time to first immobilization (G) was also evaluated. Data are expressed as the mean ± SEM. $$p < 0.01 versus WT mice treated with morphine + nx; **p < 0.01 versus WT mice treated with saline + nx; +p < 0.05, ++p < 0.01, +++p < 0.001 versus WT mice treated with saline+nx; ##p < 0.01, ###p < 0.001 versus KO mice treated with saline + nx; &&&p < 0.001 versus WT mice treated with morphine + nx.*

important to clarify that different neural elements mediate several withdrawal behaviors [77, 78]. Thus, it is not easy to extrapolate naloxone-precipitated jumping in CRF1R KO mice to other physical symptoms like body weight loss.

4. Role of CRF1 receptor in CPA expression and extinction

It is commonly accepted that affective drug withdrawal symptoms are of major motivational significance in contributing to relapse and continued drug use; thus, it is important to understand the mechanisms that mediate affective behaviors during morphine withdrawal. CPA paradigm is a highly sensitive animal model for the measurement of the negative affective component of drug withdrawal as well as to investigate the neural substrates underlying the aversive memory associated with drug withdrawal [79, 80]. In this model, a morphine-dependent animal undergoing withdrawal is exposed to a particular environment for a period of time. When later is given the opportunity to freely explore the apparatus, animals trained in this way tend to avoid the previously paired context due to the association between the context and aversive memories of drug withdrawal [79].

The extinction of this aversion occurs if the association is weakened by repeated exposure to the withdrawal-associated context in the absence of the conditioned stimulus, and the initial response (CPA) can be reinstated by a drug priming injection, stress or by conditioned cues. Extinction is complete when animals no longer avoid the previously cue-paired compartment. Typically, while memory reconsolidation requires single context reexposure, extinction requires multiple cue reexposures [81]. For example, fear conditioning studies suggest that the extinction process does not eliminate the initial context, but the organism learns that this cue does not cause the previous stimulus [82]. Thus, extinction requires associative learning, consolidation, and the formation of a new memory [83].

Recently, our group has investigated the mechanism underlying CPA expression and extinction. These experiments showed that morphine administration induced a significant place aversion for the naloxone-paired compartment, compared to the saline group. However, CRF1R KO mice presented less aversion than wild type mice (**Figure 7A**).

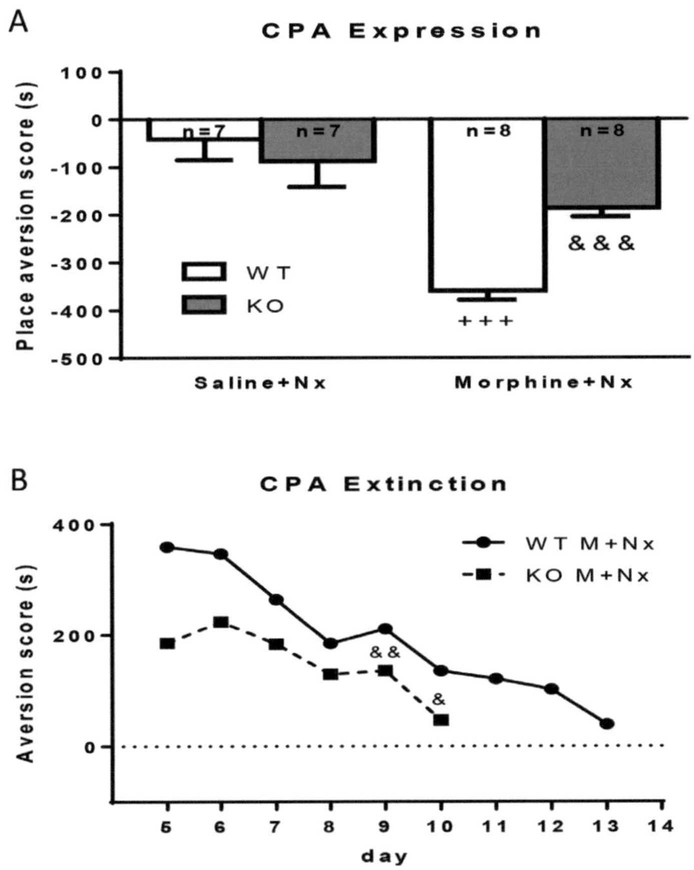

Figure 7.
(A) CPA expression induced by naloxone (nx, 1 mg/kg, s.c.) in wild type (WT) or knockout (CRF1R KO) mice treated with morphine or saline. The score was calculated for each mouse as the difference between the postconditioning and the preconditioning time spent in the naloxone-paired compartment. (B) Extinction of CPA training. Aversion scores from day 5 to 13 for WT and CRF1R KO mice are shown. Data are expressed as the mean ± SEM. +++p < 0.001 versus WT mice treated with saline + nx, &p < 0.05, &&p < 0.01, &&&p < 0.001 versus WT mice treated with morphine + nx.

There is much information about the neurobiological mechanisms involving extinction of reward memory of drug taking [84–86]. However, little information is known about extinction of aversive memory of drug withdrawal [87]. Previous studies have demonstrated that the aversive effects of opiates might be related to basal genotype differences in the brain systems [88]. Accordingly, we have clearly demonstrated that the genetic disruption of the CRF/CRF1R pathway decreases the period of CPA extinction (**Figure 7B**).

Thus, results obtained by our laboratory regarding CPA expression and extinction suggest an important role for CRF1R in aversive memory.

5. Role of HHA axis in the CPA induced by morphine withdrawal

It is well established that acute withdrawal of all major drugs of abuse dysregulates the HPA axis and alters CRF activity in the PVN of the hypothalamus, with a common response of increased adrenocorticotropic hormone (ACTH) and corticosterone [89], which mediate somatic and aversive components of withdrawal [72, 90–92]. To evaluate whether a causal link exists between CRF1R activation and HPA axis, our group has measured plasma ACTH and corticosterone levels in wild type and CRF1R KO mice after naloxone-induced CPA expression and CPA extinction (**Figure 8**). Our investigations have shown that plasma ACTH levels are increased in wild type mice although plasma corticosterone levels are not changed following CPA expression. These results indicate that ACTH-independent mechanisms could have an important role in the regulation of the adrenal stress system to appropriately adapt its response to physiological necessities, and even the presence of pituitary ACTH is basic for adrenocortical function. Numerous lines of evidence indicate that a large number of neuropeptides, neurotransmitters, growth

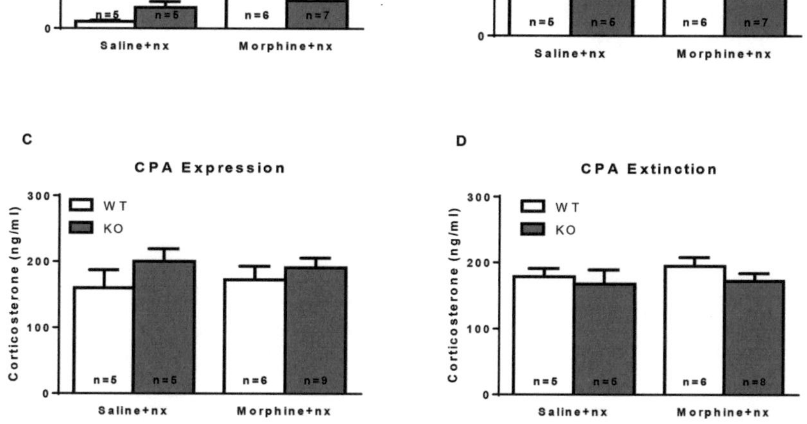

Figure 8.
Effect of CPA expression and CPA extinction training on ACTH (A and B) and corticosterone (C and D) plasma levels in wild type (WT) and knockout (CRF1R KO) mice. Data are expressed as the mean ± SEM. +++p < 0.001 versus WT mice treated with saline + nx, &&&p < 0.001 versus WT mice treated with morphine + nx.

factors, and bacterial ligands can influence the release of adrenal glucocorticoids independently of pituitary ACTH [93]. Adrenocortical cells express a large diversity of receptors for these factors, thus triggering potential direct actions on glucocorticoids release. Damage in the upstream stress regulating pathways in the brain leads to a rupture between ACTH and corticosterone, which suggests that central nervous system neurocircuits can regulate HPA axis response at both pituitary and adrenal sites [94]. Our results also indicate that CPA expression-induced ACTH release is attenuated in CRF1R KO mice. In agreement with these observations, it has been reported fewer ACTH levels in morphine withdrawn animals treated with CRF1R antagonists [70]. Besides, a role for the HPA axis and extra-hypothalamic brain circuitry in somatic, molecular, and endocrine changes induced during opioid withdrawal has been described [72]. ACTH plasma levels returned to basal in wild type and CRF1R KO mice after CPA extinction. These results suggest that CPA expression is, at least, partially due to an increase in plasma ACTH levels which can be decreased after naloxone CPA extinction.

6. Conclusion

CP-154,526 administration or genetic deletion of CRF1R impairs CPP and CPA learning, suggesting that the expression of reward and aversive learning and memory shares some common neural circuits related with CRF/CRF1R signaling. During the formation or consolidation process (CPP expression), the majority of phospho-CREB positive neurons in DG coexpresses Trx-1, in parallel with an increased expression of BDNF, suggesting that Trx-1 could activate CREB and this in turn accelerates the transcription of CREB-dependent genes such as BDNF. However, CP-154,526 diminishes CPP expression, in parallel with a block of phospho-CREB/Trx-1 colocalization and BDNF expression, suggesting that Trx-1-CREB-BDNF signaling could be essential for memory formation or consolidation. In addition, CPA expression training increases plasma ACTH levels, which is critical for the maintenance of aversive memories associated with drug withdrawal. Genetic deletion of CRF1R (KO mice) induces a reduction in CPA expression accompanied with a higher decrease in ACTH plasma levels. CPA extinction period is reduced in KO mice, indicating a role for CRF1R in the aversive memory retrieval. Altogether, these results indicate a critical role for CRF, through CRF1R, in molecular changes involved in reward memory-associated behaviors and in aversive memory expression and extinction. The disruption of these processes by CRF1 antagonists might lead to effective treatments in drug addiction.

Acknowledgements

This research was supported by a grant from the Ministerio de Economía, Industria y Competitividad (SAF2017-85679-R).

Author details

Pilar Almela*, Juan A. García-Carmona, Elena Martínez-Laorden, María V. Milanés and María L. Laorden
Department of Pharmacology, Faculty of Medicine, University of Murcia, Murcia, Spain

*Address all correspondence to: palmela@um.es

References

[1] Leshner AI. Drug abuse and addiction treatment research. The next generation. Archives of General Psychiatry. 1997;**54**:691-694

[2] O'Brien CP, Childress AR, McLellan AT, Ehrman R. Classical conditioning in drug-dependent humans. Annals of the New York Academy of Sciences. 1992;**654**:400-415

[3] O'Brien CP, McLellan AT. Myths about the treatment of addiction. Lancet. 1996;**347**:237-240

[4] Childers A, Ehrman R, McLellan AT, O'Brien C. Conditioned craving and arousal in cocaine addiction: A preliminary report. NIDA Research Monograph. 1988;**81**:74-80

[5] Tzschentke TM. Measuring reward with the conditioned place preference (CPP) paradigm: Update of the last decade. Addiction Biology. 2007;**12**:227-462. DOI: 10.1111/j.1369-1600.2007.00070.x

[6] Childs E, de Wit H. Amphetamine-induced place preference in humans. Biological Psychiatry. 2009;**65**:900-904. DOI: 10.1016/j.biopsych.2008.11.016

[7] Childs E, de Wit H. Contextual conditioning enhances the psychostimulant and incentive properties of d-amphetamine in humans. Addiction Biology. 2013;**18**:985-992. DOI: 10.1111/j.1369-1600.2011.00416.x

[8] Martin del Campo AF, McMurray RG, Besser GM, Grossman A. Effect of 12-hour infusion of naloxone on mood and cognition in normal male volunteers. Biological Psychiatry. 1992;**32**:344-353. DOI: 10.1016/0006-3223(92)90038-2

[9] LaLumiere RT, Kalivas PW. Glutamate release in the nucleus accumbens core is necessary for heroin seeking. The Journal of Neuroscience. 2008;**28**:3170-3177. DOI: 10.1523/JNEUROSCI.5129-07

[10] Lee AM, Messing RO. Protein kinases and addiction. Annals of the New York Academy of Sciences. 2008;**1141**:22-57. DOI: 10.1196/annals.1441.022

[11] Ron D, Jurd R. The 'ups and downs' of signaling cascades in addiction. Science's STKE. 2005;**2005**:re14. DOI: 10.1126/stke.3092005re14

[12] Russo SJ, Mazei-Robison MS, Ables JL, Nestler EJ. Neurotrophic factors and structural plasticity in addiction. Neuropharmacology. 2009;**56**(Suppl 1):73-82. DOI: 10.1016/j.neuropharm.2008.06.059

[13] Wise RA. Dopamine and reward: The anhedonia hypothesis 30 years on. Neurotoxicity Research. 2008;**14**: 169-183. DOI: 10.1007/BF03033808

[14] Chen Y, Bender RA, Brunson KL, Pomper JK, Grigoriadis DE, Wurst W, et al. Modulation of dendritic differentiation by corticotropin-releasing factor in the developing hippocampus. PNAS. 2004;**101**:15782-15787. DOI: 10.1073/pnas.0403975101

[15] Korosi A, Veening JG, Kozicz T, Henckens M, Dederen J, Groenink L. Distribution and expression of CRF receptor 1 and 2 mRNAs in the CRF over-expressing mouse brain. Brain Research. 2006;**1072**:46-55. DOI: 10.1016/j.brainres.2005.12.034

[16] Lim MM, Tsivkovskaia NO, Bai Y, Young LJ, Ryabinin AE. Distribution of corticotropin-releasing factor and urocortin 1 in the vole brain. Brain, Behavior and Evolution. 2006;**68**: 229-240. DOI: 10.1159/000094360

[17] Refojo D, Echenique C, Muller MB, Reul JM, Deussing JM, Wurst W, et al. Corticotropin-releasing hormone activates ERK1/2MAPK in specific brain areas. PNAS. 2005;**102**:6183-6188. DOI: 10.1073/pnas.0502070102

[18] García-Carmona JA, Almela P, Baroja-Mazo A, Milanés MV, Laorden ML. Restricted role of CRF1R for the activity of brainstem catecholaminergic neurons in the negative state of morphine withdrawal. Psychopharmacology. 2012;**220**:379-393. DOI: 10.1007/s00213-011-2478-y

[19] Haass-Koffler CL, Bartlett SE. Stress and addiction: Contribution of the corticotropin releasing factor (CRF) system in neuroplasticity. Frontiers in Molecular Neuroscience. 2012;**5**:1-13. DOI: 10.3389/fnmol.2012.00091

[20] Vivar C, van Praag H. Functional circuits of new neurons in the dentate gyrus. Neural Circuits. 2013;**7**:1-13. DOI: 10.3389/fncir.2013.00015

[21] Chen Y, Bender RA, Frotscer M, Baram TZ. Novel and transient populations of corticotropin-releasing hormone-expressing neurons in developing hippocampus suggest unique functional roles: A quantitative spatiotemporal analysis. The Journal of Neuroscience. 2001;**21**:7171-7181

[22] Kasagi Y, Horiba N, Sakai K, Fukuda Y, Suda T. Involvement of cAMP-response element binding protein in corticotropin-releasing factor (CRF)-induced down-regulation of CRF receptor 1 gene expression in rat anterior pituitary cells. Journal of Neuroendocrinology. 2002;**14**:587-592

[23] Briand LA, Lee BG, Lelay J, Kaestner KH, Blendy JA. Serine 133 phosphorylation is not required for hippocampal CREB-mediated transcription and behavior. Learning & Memory. 2015;**22**:109-115. DOI: 10.1101/lm.037044.114

[24] Dallman MF, Akana SF, Strack AM, Hanson ES, Sebastian RJ. The neural network that regulates energy balance is responsive to glucocorticoids and insulin and also regulates HPA axis responsivity at a site proximal to CRF neurons. Annals of the New York Academy of Sciences. 1995;**771**:730-742

[25] Martín F, Laorden ML, Milanés MV. Morphine withdrawal regulates phosphorylation of cAMP response element binding protein (CREB) through PKC in the nucleus tractus solitarius-A2 catecholaminergic neurons. Journal of Neurochemistry. 2009;**110**:1422-1432. DOI: 10.1111/j.1471-4159.2009.06234

[26] Martín F, Mora L, Laorden ML, Milanés MV. Protein kinase C phosphorylates the cAMP response element binding protein in the hypothalamic paraventricular nucleus during morphine withdrawal. British Journal of Pharmacology. 2011;**163**:857-875. DOI: 10.1111/j.1476-5381.2011.01287.x

[27] Voorn P, Jorritsma-Byham B, Van Dijk C, Buijs RM. The dopaminergic innervation of the ventral striatum in the rat: A light- and electron-microscopical study with antibodies against dopamine. The Journal of Comparative Neurology. 1986;**251**: 84-99. DOI: 10.1002/cne.902510106

[28] Séguéla P, Watkins KC, Descarries L. Ultrastructural features of dopamine axon terminals in the anteromedial and the suprarhinal cortex of adult rat. Brain Research. 1988;**442**:11-22

[29] García-Carmona JA, Milanés MV, Laorden ML. Brain stress system response after morphine-conditioned place preference. The International Journal of Neuropsychopharmacology. 2013;**10**:1-13. DOI: 10.1017/S1461145713000588

[30] García-Carmona JA, Camejo DM, Almela P, Jiménez A, Milanés MV,

Sevilla F, Laorden ML. CP-154,526 modifies CREB phosphorylation and thioredoxin-1 expression in the dentate gyrus following morphine-induced conditioned place preference. PLoS One. 2015;**10**(8):e0136164. DOI: 10.1371/journal.pone.0136164

[31] González-Cuello A, Mora L, Hidalgo JM, Meca N, Lasheras C, Milanés MV, Laorden ML. Enhanced tyrosine hydroxylase phosphorylation in the nucleus accumbens and nucleus tractus solitarius-A2 cell group after morphine-conditioned place preference. Naunyn-Schmiedeberg's Archives of Pharmacology. 2010;**382**:525-534. DOI: 10.1007/s00210-010-0567-9

[32] Lasheras MC, Laorden ML, Milanés MV, Núñez C. Corticotropin-releasing factor 1 receptor mediates the activity of the reward system evoked by morphine-induced conditioned place preference. Neuropharmacology. 2015;**95**:168-180. DOI: 10.1016/j.neuropharm.2014.12.021

[33] Ma YY, Meng L, Guo CHY, Han JS, Lee D, Cui CL. Dose- and time-dependent, context-induced elevation of dopamine and its metabolites in the nucleus accumbens of morphine-induced CPP rats. Behavioural Brain Research. 2009;**204**:192-199. DOI: 10.1016/j.bbr.2009.06.017

[34] Zarrindast MR, Ebrahimi-Ghiri M, Rostami P, Rezayof A. Repeated pre-exposure to morphine into the ventral pallidum enhances morphine-induced place preference: Involvement of dopaminergic and opioidergic mechanisms. Behavioural Brain Research. 2007;**181**:35-41. DOI: 10.1016/j.bbr.2007.03.019

[35] Ewan EE, Martin TJ. Rewarding electrical brain stimulation in rats after peripheral nerve injury: Decreased facilitation by commonly abused prescription opioids. Anesthesiology. 2011;**115**:1271-1280. DOI: 10.1097/ALN.0b013e3182330448

[36] Rodaros D, Caruana DA, Amir S, Stewart J. Corticotropin-releasing factor projections from limbic forebrain and paraventricular nucleus of the hypothalamus to the region of the ventral tegmental area. Neuroscience. 2007;**105**:8-13. DOI: 10.1016/j.neuroscience.2007.09.043

[37] Chen YW, Rada PV, Bützler BP, Leibowitz SF, Hoebel BG. Corticotropin releasing factor in the nucleus accumbens shell induces swim depression, anxiety, and anhedonia along with changes in local dopamine/acetyl-choline balance. Neuroscience. 2012;**206**:155-166. DOI: 10.1016/j.neuroscience.2011.12.009

[38] Ewan EE, Martin TJ. Analgesics as reinforcers with chronic pain: Evidence from operant studies. Neuroscience Letters. 2013;**557**(Pt A):60-64. DOI: 10.1016/j.neulet.2013.08.018

[39] Nestler EJ. Common molecular and cellular substrates of addiction and memory. Neurobiology of Learning and Memory. 2002;**73**:637-647. DOI: 10.1006/nlme.2002.4084

[40] Zhou LF, Zhu YP. Changes of CREB in rat hippocampus, prefrontal cortex and nucleus accumbens during three phases of morphine induced conditioned place preference in rats. Journal of Zhejiang University. Science. B. 2006;**7**:107-113. DOI: 10.1631/jzus.2006.B0107

[41] Moron JA, Gullapalli S, Taylor C, Gupta A, Gomes I, Deve LA. Modulation of opiate-related signalling molecules in morphine-dependent conditioned behaviour: Conditioned place preference to morphine induces CREB phosphorylation. Neuropsychopharmacology. 2010;**35**:955-966. DOI: 10.1038/npp.2009.199

[42] Walters CL, Blendy JA. Different requirements for cAMP response

element binding protein in positive and negative reinforcing properties of drugs of abuse. The Journal of Neuroscience. 2001;**21**:9438-9444

[43] Koob GF. A role of brain stress system in addiction. Neuron. 2008;**59**:11-34. DOI: 10.1016/j.neuron.2008.06.012

[44] Von Wolff G, Avrabos CH, Stepan J, Wurst W, Deussing JM, Holsboer F, Eder M. Voltage-sensitive dye imaging demonstrated an enhancing effect of corticotropin-releasing hormone on neuronal activity propagation through the hippocampal formation. Journal of Psychiatric Research. 2011;**45**:256-261. DOI: 10.1016/j.jpsychires.2010.06.007

[45] Gonzalo-Ruiz A, Morte L, Flecha JM, Sanz JM. Neurotransmitter characteristics of neurons projecting to the suprammamillary nucleus of the rat. Anatomy and Embryology (Berlin). 1999;**200**:377-392

[46] Choi WK, Wirtshafter D, Park HJ, Lee MS, Her S, Shim I. The characteristics of supramammillary cells projecting to the hippocampus in stress response in rat. The Korean Journal of Physiology & Pharmacology. 2012;**16**:17-24. DOI: 10.4196/kjpp.2012.16.1.17

[47] Wiesner B, Roloff B, Fechner K, Slominski A. Intracellular calcium measurements of single human skin cells after stimulation with corticotropin-releasing factor and urocortin using confocal laser scanning microscopy. Journal of Cell Science. 2003;**116**:1261-1268. DOI: 10.1242/jcs.00301

[48] Fazal N, Slominski A, Choudhry MA, Wei ET, Sayeed MM. Effect of CRF and related peptides on calcium signaling in human and rodent melanoma cells. FEBS Letters. 1998;**435**:187-190. DOI: 10.1016/S0014-5793(98)01067-9

[49] Pisarchik A, Slominski A. Molecular and functional characterization of novel CRFR1 isoforms from the skin. European Journal of Biochemistry. 2004;**27**:2821-2830. DOI: 10.1111/j.1432-1033.2004.04216.x

[50] Zbytek B, Pfeffer LM, Slominski AT. Corticotropin-releasing hormone stimulates NF-kappaB in human epidermal keratinocytes. The Journal of Endocrinology. 2004;**181**:R1-R7

[51] Zbytek B, Slominski AT. Corticotropin-releasing hormone induces keratinocyte differentiation in the adult human epidermis. Journal of Cellular Physiology. 2005;**203**:118-126. DOI: 10.1002/jcp.20209

[52] Zmijewski MA, Slominski AT. CRF1 receptor splicing in epidermal keratinocytes: Potential biological role and environmental regulations. Journal of Cellular Physiology. 2009;**218**: 593-602. DOI: 10.1002/jcp.21632

[53] Inda C, Armando NG, Dos Santos Claro PA, Silberstein S. Endocrinology and the brain: Corticotropin-releasing hormone signalling. Endocrine Connections. 2017;**6**:R99-R120. DOI: 10.1530/EC-17-0111

[54] Hirota K, Matsui M, Murata M, Takashima Y, Cheng FS, et al. Nucleoredoxin, glutaredoxin and thioredoxin differentially regulate NF-kB, AP-1 and CREB activation in HEK293 cells. Biochemical and Biophysical Research Communications. 2000;**274**:177-182. DOI: 10.1006/bbrc.2000.3106

[55] Luo FC, Qi L, Lv T, Wang SD, Liu H, et al. Geranylgeranylacetone protects mice against morphine induced hyperlocomotion, rewarding effect, and withdrawal syndrome. Free Radical Biology & Medicine. 2012;**52**:1218-1227. DOI: 10.1016/j.freeradbiomed.2012.01.004

[56] Lv T, Wang SD, Bai J. Thioredoxin-1 was required for CREB activity by methamphetamine in rat pheochromocytoma cells. Cellular and Molecular Neurobiology. 2013;**33**:319-325. DOI: 10.1007/s10571-012-9897-0

[57] Luo FC, Feng YM, Zhao L, Kui L, Wang SD, Song JY, et al. Thioredoxin-1 expression regulated by morphine in sh-sy5y cells. Neuroscience Letters. 2012;**523**:50-55. DOI: 10.1016/j.neulet.2012.06.039

[58] Kondo N, Nakamura H, Masutani H, Yodoi J. Redox regulation of human thioredoxin network. Antioxidants & Redox Signaling. 2006;**8**:1881-1890. DOI: 10.1089/ars.2006.8.1881

[59] Franklin KBJ, Paxinos G. The Mouse Brain in Stereotaxic Coordinates. 3rd ed. San Diego: Academic Press; 2008. p. 256

[60] Jia JJ, Zeng XS, Li Y, Ma S, Bai J. Ephedrine induced thioredoxin-1 expression through β-adrenergic receptor/cyclic AMP/protein kinase A/dopamine-and cyclic AMP-regulated phosphoprotein signaling pathway. Cellular Signalling. 2013;**25**:1194-1201. DOI: 10.1016/j.cellsig.2013.02.007

[61] Zhong P, Liu Y, Hu Y, Wang T, Zhao YP, Liu QS. BDNF interacts with endocannabinoids to regulate cocaine-induced synaptic plasticity in mouse midbrain dopamine neurons. The Journal of Neuroscience. 2015;**35**:4469-4481. DOI: 10.1523/JNEUROSCI.2924-14

[62] Lv XF, Sun LL, Cui CL, Han JS. Nac shell Arc/Arg3.1 protein mediates reconsolidation of morphine CPP by increased GluR1 cell surface expression: Activation of ERK-coupled CREB is required. The International Journal of Neuropsychopharmacology. 2015;**18**:pyv030. DOI: 10.1093/ijnp/pyv030

[63] Kandel ER. The molecular biology of memory storage: A dialog between genes and synapses. Bioscience Reports. 2001;**21**:565-611. DOI: 10.1126/science.1067020

[64] Barco A, Alarcon JM, Kandel ER. Expression of constitutively active CREB protein facilitates the late phase of long-term potentiation by enhancing synaptic capture. Cell. 2002;**108**:689-703. DOI: 10.1016/S0092-8674(02)00657-8

[65] Bramham CR, Messaoudi E. BDNF function in adult synaptic plasticity: The synaptic consolidation hypothesis. Progress in Neurobiology. 2005;**76**:99-125. DOI: 10.1016/j.pneurobio.2005.06.003

[66] Alvandi MS, Bourmpoula M, Homberg JR, Fathollahi Y. Association of contextual cues with morphine reward increases neural and synaptic plasticity in the ventral hippocampus of rats. Addiction Biology. 2017;**22**:1883-1894. DOI: 10.1111/adb.12547

[67] Wan L, Xie Y, Su L, Liu Y, Wang Y, Wang Z. Rack1 affects morphine reward via BDNF. Brain Research. 2011;**1416**:26-34. DOI: 10.1016/j.brainres.2011.07.045

[68] Radke AK, Hotz NA, Gewirtz ME, Carroll ME. Reduced emotional signs of opiate withdrawal in rats selectively bred for low (LoS) versus high (HiS) saccharin intake. Psychopharmacology. 2013;**227**:117-126. DOI: 10.1007/s00213-012-2945-0

[69] García-Carmona JA, Almela P, Baroja-Mazo A, Milanés MV, Laorden ML. Restricted role of CRF1 receptor for the activity of brainstem catecholaminergic neurons in the negative state of morphine withdrawal. Psychopharmacology. 2012;**220**:379-393. DOI: 10.1007/s00213-011-2478-y

[70] Navarro-Zaragoza J, Núñez C, Laorden ML, Milanés MV. Effects of corticotropin-releasing factor receptor-1 antagonists on the brain stress system

response to morphine withdrawal. Molecular Pharmacology. 2010;**77**: 864-873. DOI: 10.1124/mol.109.062463

[71] Iredale PA, Alvaro JD, Lee Y, Terwilliger R, Chen YL, Duman RS. Role of corticotropin-releasing factor receptor-1 in opiate withdrawal. Journal of Neurochemistry. 2000;**74**:199-208. DOI: 10.1046/j.1471-4159.2000.0740199.x

[72] Papaleo F, Kitchener P, Contarino A. Disruption of the CRF/CRF1 receptor stress system exacerbates the somatic signs of opiate withdrawal. Neuron. 2007;**53**:577-589. DOI: 10.1016/j.neuron.2007.01.022

[73] Blum K, Eubanks JD, Wiggins B, Wallace JE. Morphine withdrawal reactions in male and female mice. The American Journal of Drug and Alcohol Abuse. 1976;**3**:363-368

[74] El-Kadi AO, Sharif SI. The influence of various experimental conditions on the expression of naloxone-induced withdrawal symptoms in mice. General Pharmacology. 1994;**25**:1505-1510

[75] Miyamoto Y, Takemori AE. Relative involvement of supraspinal and spinal mu opioid receptors in morphine dependence in mice. Life Sciences. 1993;**52**:1039-1044

[76] Way EL, Lou HH, Shen FH. Simultaneous quantitative assessment of morphine tolerance and physical dependence. The Journal of Pharmacology and Experimental Therapeutics. 1969;**167**:1-8

[77] Brandao ML. Involvement of opioid mechanisms in the dorsal periaqueductal gray in drug abuse. Reviews in the Neurosciences. 1993;**4**:397-405

[78] Koob GF, Maldonado R, Stinus L. Neural substrates of opiate withdrawal. Trends in Neurosciences. 1992;**15**:186-191

[79] Myers KM, Bechtholt-Gompf AJ, Coleman BR, Carlezon WA. Extinction of conditioned opiate withdrawal in rats in a two-chambered place conditioning apparatus. Nature Protocols. 2012;**7**: 517-526. DOI: 10.1038/nprot.2011.458

[80] Stinus L, Caille S, Koob GF. Opiate withdrawal-induced place aversion lasts for up to 16 weeks. Psychopharmacology. 2000;**149**:115-120

[81] Power AE, Berlau DJ, McGaugh JL, Steward O. Anisomycin infused into the hippocampus fails to block "reconsolidation" but impairs extinction: The role of re-exposure duration. Learning & Memory. 2006;**13**:27-34. DOI: 10.1101/lm.91206

[82] Bouton ME. Context and behavioral processes in extinction. Learning & Memory. 2004;**11**:485-494. DOI: 10.1101/lm.78804

[83] Milad MR, Quirk GJ. Neurons in medial prefrontal cortex signal memory for fear extinction. Nature. 2002;**420**:70-74. DOI: 10.1038/nature01138

[84] Feltenstein MW, See RE. NMDA receptor blockade in the basolateral amygdala disrupts consolidation of stimulus-reward memory and extinction learning during reinstatement of cocaine-seeking in an animal model of relapse. Neurobiology of Learning and Memory. 2007;**88**: 435-444. DOI: 10.1016/j.nlm.2007.05.006

[85] Hsu E, Packard MG. Medial prefrontal cortex infusions of bupivacaine or AP-5 block extinction of amphetamine conditioned place preference. Neurobiology of Learning and Memory. 2008;**89**:504-512. DOI: 10.1016/j.nlm.2007.08.006

[86] Torregrossa MM, Sanchez H, Taylor JR. D-cycloserine reduces the context specificity of pavlovian extinction of

cocaine cues through actions in the nucleus accumbens. The Journal of Neuroscience. 2010;**30**:10526-10533. DOI: 10.1523/JNEUROSCI.2523-10.2010

[87] Myers KM, Carlezon WA Jr. D-cycloserine facilitates extinction of naloxone-induced conditioned place aversion in morphine-dependent rats. Biological Psychiatry. 2010;**67**:85-87. DOI: 10.1016/j.biopsych.2009.08.015

[88] Solecki W, Turek A, Kubik J, Przewlocki R. Motivational effects of opiates in conditioned place preference and aversion paradigm-a study in three inbred strains of mice. Psychopharmacology. 2009;**207**:245-255. DOI: 10.1007/s00213-009-1672-7

[89] Ueno K, Maeda T, Kiguchi N, Kobayashi Y, Ozaki M, Kishioka S. Availability of serum corticosterone level for quantitative evaluation of morphine withdrawal in mice. Drug Discoveries & Therapeutics. 2011;**5**:71-75. DOI: 10.5582/ddt.2011.v5.2.71

[90] Contarino A, Papaleo F. The corticotropin-releasing factor receptor-1 pathway mediates the negative affective states of opiate withdrawal. Proceedings of the National Academy of Sciences of the United States of America. 2005;**102**:18649-18654. DOI: 10.1073/pnas.0506999102

[91] Harris GC, Aston-Jones G. Activation in extended amygdale corresponds to alter hedonic processing during protracted morphine withdrawal. Behavioural Brain Research. 2007;**176**:251-258. DOI: 10.1016/j.bbr.2006.10.012

[92] Koob GF. A role for brain stress system in addiction. Neuron. 2008;**59**:11-34. DOI: 10.1016/j.neuron.2008.06.012

[93] Bornstein SR, Engeland WC, Ehrhart-Bornstein ME, Herman JP. Dissociation of ACTH and glucocorticoids. Trends in Endocrinology and Metabolism. 2008;**19**:175-180. DOI: 10.1016/j.tem.2008.01.009

[94] Choi DC, Furai AR, Evanson NK, Ostrander MM, Ulrich-Lai YM, Herman JP. Bed nucleus of the stria terminalis subregions differentially regulates hypothalamic-pituitary-adrenal axis activity: Implications for the integration of limbic inputs. The Journal of Neuroscience. 2007;**27**:2025-2034. DOI: 10.1523/JNEUROSCI.4301-06.2007

Chapter 6

Present and Future Pharmacological Treatments for Opioid Addiction

Maria Carmen Blanco-Gandía, Sandra Montagud-Romero and Marta Rodríguez-Arias

Abstract

When treating opioid addiction, multidisciplinary treatment is highly recommended, but pharmacotherapy plays a key role. Although the ideal goal is to achieve complete abstinence, an elevated percentage of opioid addicts requires maintenance substitution therapy. In the first section of this chapter, we will focus on the current pharmacological interventions to treat opioid addiction, such as methadone, buprenorphine, and naltrexone. Thanks to these medications, people are able to go back to their normal lives, by preventing withdrawal symptoms, reducing craving, and increasing their adherence to psychotherapy. In the second section, based on the evidence that addiction induces neuroadaptive changes in several neurotransmission systems, we focus on the wide range of possible pharmacological developments at the preclinical and clinical levels, which in recent years have increased considerably.

Keywords: opioid, methadone, buprenorphine, naltrexone, naloxone

1. Introduction

Addiction is a chronic and multifactorial disorder characterized by compulsive drug seeking and use, despite its harmful consequences. Chronic opioid use induces profound molecular and behavioral changes, inducing long-lasting changes in brain plasticity [1]. During the use of the drug, reward and motivation circuits are modified, and new learning and memories are created in relation to the pleasurable effects of the drug and the context in which it is consumed [2]. These memories will later be responsible for the vulnerability to relapse even after a long period of withdrawal. In order to restructure these memories and avoid relapse and craving to opioids, the first recommended approach currently consists in combining psychotherapy with pharmacological substitution therapy [3]. Opioid addiction is currently a major medical and social problem, and its abuse and recreational use have been declared an epidemic in the USA [4, 5], with more than 90 people dying from an opioid overdose every day [6].

Opioids are highly addictive because they induce euphoria (positive reinforcement) and the cessation of a chronic use produces dysphoria [7]. The non-medical opioid use is a major public health challenge, making opioids the second most used illicit drug in the USA [8].

IntechOpen

The use of opioids has increased 10- to 14-fold in the last 20 years, including those taken under supervision and recreational use [9].

In relation to this, opioids are one of the most commonly misused medications. Although it is usually prescribed to treat pain, its abuse has serious medical consequences. According to NIDA (National Institute on Drug Abuse, NIH), misuse of prescription drugs is defined as taking a medication in a manner or dose different than has been prescribed, either for a medical complaint, such as pain, or to feel euphoria [2]. The number of opioid prescriptions has increased significantly since the early 1990s [10], with this easier access to the drug being one of the reasons for the high prevalence of opioid misuse [9]. However, other factors can contribute to the problem, such as the lack of information about the addictive properties of prescription opioids, which are perceived as less harmful than illicit opioids [11, 12]. Regardless of the primary causes, there has been a dramatic increase in the number of treatment admissions for addictive disorders related to prescription opioids, as well as the associated overdose deaths in the past 15 years [8, 13, 14].

Pharmacological treatments are essential for initiating and sustaining effective patient-, public health, and system-level interventions to reduce opioid-related morbidity and mortality [15]. In the specific case of opioid use disorders, pharmacotherapy is strongly recommended as a part of an integrated approach, also including psychosocial interventions, psychotherapy, or relapse prevention programs [16]. Until the 1960s, the opioid addiction treatment was only oriented towards abstinence, but then the potential action of methadone as a maintenance treatment for opioid addiction was evaluated [17]. Currently, although complete abstinence continues to be the best possible outcome, the most common option is life-long substitution therapy. While the currently approved medications improve the outcomes, relapse rates are still high, and pharmacotherapy is not effective in all patients [18].

The final goal of the treatment is to reduce the risk of illicit opioid use, overdose or infections, as well as the general improvement of the individuals' quality of life [15]. The available pharmacological interventions prevent the appearance of withdrawal symptoms and reduce craving, also increasing adherence to the psychotherapy. First, we will address the three different approved drugs on the market [19]. Although the rate of success, measured by maintenance of abstinence, has been greatly improved with the existing treatments, there is still room for further improvement. In a second part of this chapter, we will also refer to new treatments under development, both in preclinical models and in clinical trials. These new drugs are focused on different neurotransmission systems, which are altered by the neuroadaptive changes induced during the addictive process.

2. Current approved pharmacological treatments for opioid addiction

2.1 Opioid agonist therapies

The great percentage of withdrawn patients who relapse into drug use [20] makes opioid maintenance therapy the first-line treatment in most cases. Ideal agents for substitution maintenance therapy are those with a high affinity for μ-type opioid receptors showing long-term action. Methadone and buprenorphine, as potent and long-acting opioid agonists, are usually prescribed for opioid substitution therapy, and both constitute the most effective treatments for opioid dependence [21].

2.1.1 Methadone

Methadone is a safe, efficient, and effective treatment for heroin addiction [22]. This μ-opioid receptor agonist was introduced in the USA by Eli Lilly and Company as an opioid analgesic in 1947. Methadone maintenance treatment began at the Rockefeller Hospital (1965) with the aim to develop an effective and long action pharmacotherapy that targeted opioid receptors. In these initial clinical trials, patients received safe doses (20–40 mg) once a day, and over time, the dose was adjusted to avoid withdrawal symptoms and reduce craving [17]. Since 1964, a great number of studies have documented the safety, efficacy, and effectiveness of methadone pharmacotherapy for heroin addiction [22].

The National Institutes of Health (NIH) at the end of the 1990s supported methadone maintenance pharmacotherapy for heroin addiction. Nowadays, half of the problematic opiate users are under maintenance treatment, with more than 60% receiving methadone [23]. Elevated retention rates with a noteworthy decrease of illicit opiate use have been observed under methadone maintenance treatment [24–27]. In addition, there are reductions of other associated problems such as intravenous drug use, crime [28–30], and improvement of social functioning [31]. Later studies reported that prolonged methadone maintenance normalized the immune system function in heroin addicts [32], as well as the altered stress response [33]. Methadone is also well suited with performance of complex cognitive tasks [34]. Regarding its efficacy, according to a recent Cochrane meta-analysis, methadone and buprenorphine appear to be equally effective [35].

Regardless of the positive effects of methadone, one of the main difficulties of methadone maintenance treatment is the stigma accompanying the methadone clinics. In order to solve this, maintenance programs aim to rehabilitate patients by reassigning addicts from a traditional clinic to a medical office for ongoing treatment. The concept of medical maintenance carefully emulates the treatment of chronic diseases, such as insulin-dependent diabetes [32].

On the other hand, there are specific drug interactions of methadone [36], for example, the antituberculosis agent rifampin or the anticonvulsant phenytoin [37–39]. Methadone can also inhibit gonadotropin-releasing hormones, lowering testosterone levels [40, 41]. Finally, another recognized effect of methadone is the QT prolongation [42]. Patients who undergo prolonged QT intervals must switch to a treatment with buprenorphine, which does not affect it [43]. Several countries, including Germany and Austria, have alternative treatments for opioid maintenance, such as Levomethadone (purified methadone) [44], which exerts its pharmacologic effects mainly via agonism of μ-opioid receptor.

2.1.2 Buprenorphine

Buprenorphine and the combination buprenorphine-naloxone were also introduced as a possible treatment for opioid use disorder. This medication is characterized by a better side effect profile, lower abuse potential, and good availability when compared to methadone [3]. Buprenorphine is a μ-receptor partial agonist that can reduce opiate cravings, prevent opiate withdrawal, but at the same time blocks the effects of other more powerful opiates [45]. As partial agonist, buprenorphine presents a safety profile with respect to other μ-opioid-receptor agonists and can be more easily adjusted to the desired effect [46]. Although buprenorphine can be the first-line medication over methadone to treat opioid addiction, as it has considerable less abuse potential, its efficacy is limited when treating severe opioid use disorders. Due to the displacement of a stronger opioid by a weaker one, buprenorphine can precipitate withdrawal symptoms [33, 47]. To increase the adherence to this treatment, patients should be at least in mild withdrawal [48].

To avoid diversion, buprenorphine is usually combined with the specific opioid antagonist, naloxone. In 2006, it was introduced in the European market as a sublingual combination tablet. Several works have established the efficacy of buprenorphine-naloxone as a maintenance medication [49–51] not only for prescription opioids but also for heroin addiction [52, 53]. Numerous meta-analyses have determined that buprenorphine produces successful results in heroin dependence, with no deficiency with respect to being abstinent of illicit opioid use [54, 55]. However, methadone was found to be superior to buprenorphine in overall treatment retention [56]. Buprenorphine therapy not only improves the overall individuals' quality of life but also decreases overcrowding in emergency departments [57, 58].

From a pharmacological point of view, buprenorphine has important advantages over methadone besides the lower risk of overdose [41, 59]. It is preferable for treatment of opioid dependence in those patients with HIV/AIDS [60, 61] and for pregnant opioid users [62]. On the other hand, when buprenorphine is combined with respiratory depressants, such as alcohol or benzodiazepines, it results in sedation, coma, or even death [63]. Furthermore, patients who do not know about the pharmacology of buprenorphine and use additional opioids seeking a "high" are at risk of an overdose when the effects of buprenorphine wear off [55, 64, 65].

2.2 Opiate antagonist therapies

The antagonist therapy blocks or reduces a biological response by binding to and blocking a receptor rather than activating it like an agonist. Naloxone and naltrexone, the opioid antagonist treatments most accepted and commonly used, prevent and reverse opioid effects by mainly blocking the μ-opioid receptor. Both are employed for quick detoxification if there is an overdose and to prevent relapse [66]. Naloxone is a short-acting non-selective opioid antagonist that reverses an opioid overdose. Overdose is a common event for those who use opioids and is the leading cause of death in this population [67, 68]. It quickly crosses the blood-brain barrier and can reverse morphine-induced respiratory depression within 1–2 min [69].

Different studies support the effectiveness of community-based naloxone training and distribution programs in reducing overdose deaths [24, 70, 71]. Naloxone is considered a safe drug to use with little probability of complications, since it has no agonistic activity at the μ-opioid receptor [23]. Since opioid abuse has been declared an epidemic in the USA [4], naloxone has been made more accessible to the relatives of opioid users, which decreases potentially fatal overdoses around 30–40% [72, 73].

Naltrexone is an opioid receptor antagonist that blocks the euphoric and reinforcing effects of opioids consumption, being mainly used for detoxification programs [74–77]. However, the main disadvantage of the use of this antagonist is the low rate of adherence to this treatment, since less than 20% of patients continue opioid antagonist treatments after several months [78]. Nevertheless, with highly motivated patients or dependent people who cannot be included in the methadone program, naltrexone maintenance therapy can be proposed as a successful approach for treating opioid addiction [79]. Furthermore, it has the advantage of not generating tolerance and/or dependency [80]. In the last years, a new intra-muscular depot formulation of naltrexone has been approved, being useful in reducing the days-of-heroin-use and relapse rate compared with a placebo [81, 82]. This depot naltrexone is taken once monthly, and several studies have shown good outcomes compared to placebo in decreasing craving in naltrexone-treated patients [83].

These extended-release naltrexone formulations address the compliance problems that are often found with oral administration [84]. However, a recent comparative study shows that the extended-release naltrexone presents more difficulties in terms of induction and ongoing care with respect to other buprenorphine products, such as the sublingual film of buprenorphine-naloxone [85].

Nevertheless, to date, the extended-release naltrexone is, together with methadone and buprenorphine, the most recommended pharmacotherapy for opioid use disorders, as it has shown superiority with respect to placebo treatment and counseling [83, 86, 87].

3. New pharmacological therapies in development of opiate addiction

Drug addiction induces significant changes in numerous neurotransmission systems [1], which became new therapeutic targets to treat opioid addiction. Therefore, new pharmacological targets are constantly being developed to improve opiate addiction treatment. This second part of the review will offer an overview of the most promising agents under development and we will also discuss the recent advances in neuroinflammation and the pharmacogenetics field.

3.1 Drugs acting on opioid receptors

With the aim of increasing the efficacy and adherence of treatments, numerous studies are testing new approaches to the currently approved medications. For example, the newest buprenorphine subdermal implant called probuphine [88], which was approved by the FDA in May 2016, is prescribed to those patients who have achieved a sustained clinical stability with low-to-moderate doses of a transmucosal buprenorphine-containing product.This implant guarantees non-fluctuating blood levels of buprenorphine continuously for 6 months improving patient compliance [89].

There is growing interest in the slow-release oral morphine (SROM), as a potential effective candidate for maintenance treatment [90–92]. This medication is given once daily, and it suits those individuals who cannot tolerate methadone, respond poorly to other available treatments, or show a prolonged QT [93–95]. However, the last Cochrane meta-analysis reported that there is not enough evidence to confirm the effectiveness of SROM for opioid maintenance, as only three inconclusive studies exist [96].

Tramadol, a reuptake inhibitor of serotonin and norepinephrine, produces a metabolite that moderately acts as a μ-opioid receptor agonist [97]. Recent clinical trials have demonstrated for tramadol the same level of treatment retention and opioid withdrawal symptom suppression as buprenorphine, suggesting that this is a promising and valuable medication [98, 99]. However, although it has been used in the management of acute withdrawal, its use for maintenance treatment as a harm reduction approach has not been assessed systematically. A recent pilot study of tramadol on long-term maintenance in patients with opioid use disorders showed that most of them were able to achieve and maintain abstinence for at least 6 months [100].

3.2 Dopaminergic compounds

It is well known that dopamine (DA) neurotransmission is a common mechanism of drugs of abuse, although the use of DA compounds has not been successful [22]. Numerous preclinical studies have tested the efficacy of different DA antagonists. Acute administration of the DA D3 receptor antagonist SB277011 reduces the reinforcing effects of different drugs of abuse and diminishes opiate withdrawal syndrome [101]. The well-known antipsychotics, aripiprazole (partial DAD2 and 5HT1A agonist and a 5HT2A antagonist) and risperidone (atypical antipsychotic), block context-dependent induced relapse. Risperidone also inhibits its reinstatement into heroin seeking due to environmental cues but fails to block relapse induced by priming doses [102]. In the same line, aripiprazole inhibits the conditioned place preference (CPP) induced by morphine [103]. An ongoing clinical trial is evaluating aripiprazole effects to prevent relapse to cocaine use in patients being treated with methadone, as they could return to cocaine consumption, even when they are involved in a drug treatment program [104].

3.3 Glutamatergic compounds

Preclinical studies show that reinstatement of morphine CPP is mainly mediated through glutamatergic neurotransmission [105]. NMDA receptors modulate nociceptive signals in conjunction with opioid receptors, and after continuous morphine treatment, both receptors suffer a desensitization, which mediate analgesic tolerance [22]. Therefore, NMDA receptor antagonists can prevent the development of morphine tolerance. Ifenprodil, an NMDA antagonist, prevents the development, maintenance, and reinstatement of morphine-induced CPP, as well as reinstatement of heroin-seeking self-administration [106].

Another well-known NMDA antagonist is memantine. Animal and human studies have shown positive results in reducing opiate withdrawal and preventing relapse [107–109]. However, clinical trials have not found significant differences in treatment retention, heroin consumption, or craving with respect to placebo [110]. Although memantine administered in combination with naltrexone can improve the emerging symptoms during the early phase of treatment, this combination did not induce significant improvement in preventing relapse [111].

The nitric oxide synthase (NOS) is a neural retrograde messenger molecule involved in several opioid effects. It has been reported that NOS upregulation takes place during the development of opioid dependence [112] and its inhibition blocks opioid dependence [113, 114]. In addition, administration of NOS inhibitors diminishes the development of morphine-induced CPP [106].

3.4 GABA compounds

Baclofen is a GABA-B receptor agonist approved for spasticity treatment, and early preclinical studies suggested that it could promote abstinence from a variety of drugs of abuse [115], such as cocaine, ethanol, nicotine, and methamphetamine [116–119]. Baclofen also reduces morphine withdrawal signs in morphine-dependent animals [120, 121] and disrupts reconsolidation of conditioned reward, facilitating the extinction of the morphine-induced CPP [122]. Assadi and coworkers [123] performed a clinical trial to evaluate the possible benefit of baclofen in the maintenance treatment of opioid addicts and found that the baclofen group presented increased treatment retention being superior to placebo in terms of opiate withdrawal syndrome and depressive symptoms.

An effective add-on therapy combined with methadone or buprenorphine is pregabalin and gabapentin, which are approved for treatment of epilepsy, neuropathic pain, or fibromyalgia [124]. These medications do not act directly on GABA receptors or transporters [125] but modulate the α2-delta subunit of calcium channels, preventing the release of neurotransmitters like glutamate [126]. Both medications prevent opioid tolerance and dependence and reduce withdrawal symptoms in humans and preclinical models [127–129].

3.5 Cholinergic compounds

Numerous studies have demonstrated that the cholinergic system is also implicated in opioid addiction, as chronic morphine administration is associated with changes in gene expression in the cholinergic system, and it increases cholinergic neurons in the laterodorsal tegmental nucleus. Administration of nicotinic antagonists reduces withdrawal symptoms in rodents [130], which suggests that nicotine receptors might be a potential pharmacotherapeutic target for opioid detoxification. Furthermore, a relatively recent study evaluated the role of the $\alpha4\beta2$ nicotinic receptors as a potential therapeutic target to treat morphine dependence [131]. A recent clinical trial has evaluated the effects of varenicline, a $\alpha4\beta2$ partial agonist and $\alpha7$ full agonist, usually employed for smoking cessation. Varenicline was effective in opioid detoxification patients, as opioid withdrawal scores decrease with respect to those patients receiving a placebo [131].

Cholinesterase inhibitors, currently used to treat Alzheimer's disease, including donepezil, rivastigmine, and galantamine, increase cholinergic activity and can be potential therapeutic targets in opioid abuse and dependence treatments [132]. Preclinical models have demonstrated that these cholinesterase inhibitors prevented morphine tolerance and attenuated the acquisition and expression of morphine CPP [133].

3.6 Cannabinoid compounds

There are many studies suggesting the potential action of the endocannabinoid system in opioid dependence [134, 135]. Cannabidiol is a natural active metabolite of the *Cannabis sativa* plant, which is currently being explored for its potential anti-addiction properties [135]. It is the second most abundant cannabinoid present in the plant [136], and interestingly, it does not bind directly to cannabinoid receptors but acts as an inverse agonist at both types CB1 and CB2 [137]. Regarding this, cannabidiol has been shown to attenuate the cue-induced reinstatement of heroin seeking [138] and reduces the rewarding properties of morphine in rodents [139]. There is currently a clinical trial examining the effects of cannabidiol on drug craving in abstinent heroin-dependent subjects (ClinicalTrial.Gov identifier: NCT02539823). In addition, cannabidiol, when combined with a potent opioid like fentanyl, is well tolerated, confirming that cannabidiol would be safe in the case of a relapse in abstinent heroin abusers [140].

3.7 Neuroinflammation

The neuroimmune response is an important but relatively poorly understood process in the development of drug addiction. Research is now setting up opportunities for the development of new pharmacotherapies targeting neuroimmune dysfunction. Opioids induce direct and indirect adaptations in the peripheral and central immune systems [141] with a clear relationship between opioid dependence and inflammatory processes [142]. Opioids, such as morphine and heroin, act directly on macrophages and lymphocytes, which produce changes in the CNS, resulting in neurotoxicity [143–145]. Preclinical models show that chronic morphine treatment increases proinflammatory cytokine levels and overactivates the glia [146, 147]. The consequences include dendrite atrophy, abnormal neurogenesis, and neurodegeneration [148]. To sum up, opioids act to generate the release of pro-inflammatory cytokines, which induce the activation of the inflammatory response, and finally, this response induces changes in the architecture and functioning of the brain. Neuroinflammation derived from opioid consumption is implicated in tolerance and dependence processes based on results obtained in animal models [149–151]. Anti-inflammatory cytokines, such as the IL-10, which are well tolerated and safe in other inflammatory diseases, could be used as pharmacotherapy in addiction [152]. For example, gabapentin upregulates the anti-inflammatory cytokine IL-10 in rats [128], thus reducing inflammation. Ibudilast prevents glial cell activation, inhibiting production of proinflammatory cytokines (IL1β, IL-6, TNF-α), and increases the secretion of anti-inflammatory mediators like IL-10 [153]. Clinical trials are currently evaluating if this medication, or other glial activation inhibitors, can prevent opioid withdrawal symptoms [154].

On the other hand, peroxisome proliferator-activated receptors (PPARs) mediate anti-inflammatory and neuroprotective processes [155]. Specifically, PPARγ is strongly implicated in reward processing and motivation [156], as they are located in VTA DA neurons and modulate DA release [157], which suggests its potential role in addiction. Currently, preclinical studies have tested the PPAR-γ agonist pioglitazone, an anti-inflammatory medication, as a treatment for opioid dependence, attenuating morphine withdrawal syndrome in rats [158].

3.8 Pharmacogenetics and epigenetics

Pharmacogenetics focuses on selecting the most adequate treatment for specific patients, based on their genetic profile and thereby increasing the therapeutic action of the medication. Its goal is the discovery of gene interactions that increase the success rate of treatments [22]. There are variants of gene-encoding proteins implicated in opioid pharmacokinetics and pharmacodynamics that make the patient respond better or worse to a specific treatment. Most studies focus on genes related to the therapeutic response to methadone and buprenorphine [159]. For example, two gene interactions are determinant for the response to methadone. First, there is the ABCB1, the gene encoding the P-glycoprotein efflux transporter, of which methadone is a substrate. People with variants of this gene (subjects with a wild-type and 61A haplotype combination or homozygous for the 61A) show lower methadone requirements. On the other hand, people with the variant 118A/A in μ-opioid receptor 1 gene (MOR1) show higher methadone requirements [160]. Regarding buprenorphine, the frequency of the gene polymorphism (SLC6A3/DAT1) allele 10 in the DA transporter is much higher in non-responder individuals [161]. These studies reveal the relevance of considering genetic variants when considering treatments with methadone or buprenorphine.

Currently, it is known that it is not only the polymorphisms that we inherit but also how they are expressed, what really matters in genetics. Epigenetics studies the reversible modifications to chromatin and their potent effects on gene expression regulation. Biochemical modifications, such as DNA methylation, histone modification, or micro-RNA expression, can change the pattern of the cell's gene expression [162]. Consequently, such epigenetic changes can modify drug efficacy and its adverse effects, being necessary to take them into account in clinical pharmacology [163]. Currently, the role of epigenetics in personalized pharmacotherapy has been under-explored [164]. This field of research has increased scientific interest in the last years, as changes in DNA methylation or histone modifications alter gene expression, which affects reward, craving, and relapse [165]. For example, in opiate addiction, several changes have been reported in the μ-opioid receptor 1 (OPRM1) gene expression due to the hypermethylation of this gene's promoter [166, 167]. Increased DNA methylation can be a predisposing factor for the vulnerability to heroin addiction or it can be a consequence of it. This is a new and exciting unexplored field that could offer promising results in future years.

4. Conclusion and future directions

Opioid addiction is a chronic relapsing brain disease, being a major medical and social problem. In the past 12 years, several countries are suffering a rise in opioid consumption, not only in its recreative use but also in opioid prescriptions and related misuse and abuse [5]. The high rate of relapse observed in opioid addicts forces the use of maintenance therapy with substitution opiates to reduce damage and to avoid the consumption of illegal opioids, such as heroin. Although the currently approved pharmacotherapies for opioid addiction are effective and encourage patients to stay in treatment, there is still much room for improvement [168]. Methadone, buprenorphine, and extended-release naltrexone are currently the most effective treatments to attenuate the illicit intake of opioids and, together with psychosocial therapy, constitute the best combination to succeed in the treatment [18]. The number of new pharmacological targets is constantly increasing, but frequently, initially promising preclinical studies result in failure in the clinical trials. However, we should be optimistic, since great advances have been made in recent years, but much remains to be improved in a disease as important and complex as opiate addiction.

Acknowledgements

This work was supported by Ministerio de Economía y Competitividad (MINECO), Dirección General de Investigación PSI2014-51847-R and PSI2017-83023-R. Instituto de Salud Carlos III, Red de Trastornos Adictivos (RTA) RD12/0028/0005 y RD16/0017/0007 and Unión Europea, Fondos FEDER "una manera de hacer Europa." We wish to thank Guillermo Chulia for his English language editing.

Conflict of interest

None.

Author details

Maria Carmen Blanco-Gandía, Sandra Montagud-Romero and Marta Rodríguez-Arias*
Unit of Research Psychobiology of Drug Dependence, Department of Psychobiology, Facultad de Psicología, Universitat de Valencia, Valencia, Spain

*Address all correspondence to: marta.rodriguez@uv.es

References

[1] Koob GF, Le Moal M. Addiction and the brain antireward system. Annual Review of Psychology. 2008;**59**:29-53

[2] National Institutes on Drug Abuse. Misuse of Prescription Drugs. Available from: https://www.drugabuse.gov/publications/research-reports/misuse-prescription-drugs [Accessed: 12 June 2018]

[3] Li X, Shorter D, Kosten TR. Buprenorphine in the treatment of opioid addiction: Opportunities, challenges and strategies. Expert Opinion in Pharmacotherapy. 2014;**15**(15):2263-2275

[4] Paulozzi L, Franklin G, Kerlikowske RG, Jones CM, Ghiya N, Popovic T. CDC grand rounds: Prescription drug overdose—A US epidemic. Morbidity and Mortality Weekly. 2012;**61**(1):10

[5] Shipton EA, Shipton EE, Shipton AJ. A review of the opioid epidemic: What do we do about it? Pain and therapy. 2018;**7**(1):23-36

[6] CDC. Drug overdose deaths in the United States continue to increase in 2015. Atlanta (GA): Centers for Disease Control and Prevention; 2016. Available from: https://www.cdc.gov/drugoverdose/epidemic/index.html [Accessed: 10 June 2018]

[7] Kolodny A, Courtwright DT, Hwang CS, Kreiner P, Eadie JL, Clark TW, et al. The prescription opioid and heroin crisis: A public health approach to an epidemic of addiction. Annual Review of Public Health. 2015;**36**:559-574

[8] Substance Abuse and Mental Health Services Administration, Center for Behavioral Health Statistics and Quality. Treatment Episode Data Set (TEDS): 2003-2013. National Admissions to Substance Abuse Treatment Services. 2015. Available from: http://www.samhsa.gov/data/sites/default/files/2013_Treatment_Episode_Data_Set_National/20-1-3_Treatment_Episode_Data_Set_National.pdf [Accessed: 12 June 2018]

[9] Manchikanti L, Fellows B, Ailinani H, Pampati V. Therapeutic use, abuse, and nonmedical use of opioids: A ten-year perspective. Pain Physician. 2010;**13**(5):401-435

[10] Centers for Disease Control and Prevention (CDC). Vital signs: Overdoses of prescription opioid pain relievers–United States, 1999-2008. Morbidity and Mortality Weekly Report. 2011;**60**(43):1487-1492

[11] Daniulaityte R, Falck R, Carlson RG. "I'm not afraid of those ones just 'cause they've been prescribed": Perceptions of risk among illicit users of pharmaceutical opioids. The International Journal on Drug Policy. 2012;**23**(5):374-384

[12] Webster PC. Oxycodone class action lawsuit filed. Canadian Medical Association Journal. 2012;**184**(7):E345-E346

[13] Jones CM, McAninch JK. Emergency department visits and overdose deaths from combined use of opioids and benzodiazepines. American Journal of Preventive Medicine. 2015;**49**(4):493-501

[14] Rudd RA, Aleshire N, Zibbell JE, Gladden RM. Increases in drug and opioid overdose deaths—United States, 2000-2014. MMWR. Morbidity and Mortality Weekly Report. 2016;**64**(50-51):1378-1382

[15] Bratberg JP. Opioids, naloxone, and beyond: The intersection of medication

safety, public health, and pharmacy. Journal of the American Pharmacists Association. 2017;**57**(2):S5-S7

[16] Dematteis M, Auriacombe M, D'Agnone O, Somaini L, Szerman N, Littlewood R, et al. Recommendations for buprenorphine and methadone therapy in opioid use disorder: A European consensus. Expert Opinion on Pharmacotherapy. 2017;**18**(18):1987-1999

[17] Dole VP, Nyswander ME, Kreek MJ. Narcotic blockade. Archives of Internal Medicine. 1966;**118**(4):304-309

[18] Volkow ND, Collins FS. The role of science in addressing the opioid crisis. New England Journal of Medicine. 2017;**377**(4):391-394

[19] Bisaga A, Mannelli P, Sullivan MA, Vosburg SK, Compton P, Woody GE, et al. Antagonists in the medical management of opioid use disorders: Historical and existing treatment strategies. The American Journal on Addictions. 2018;**27**(3):177-187

[20] Amato L, Davoli M, Minozzi S, Ferroni E, Ali R, Ferri M. Methadone at tapered doses for the management of opioid withdrawal. Cochrane Database of Systematic Reviews. 2013;**2**:1-70. Artical No: CD003409

[21] Rodríguez-Arias M, Aguilar MA, Miñarro J. Therapies in early development for the treatment of opiate addiction. Expert Opinion on Investigational Drugs. 2015;**24**:1459-1472

[22] van Dorp EL, Yassen A, Dahan A. Naloxone treatment in opioid addiction: The risks and benefits. Expert Opinion on Drug Safety. 2007;**6**(2):125-132

[23] European Monitoring Centre for Drugs and Drug Addiction. (2017). European drug report 2017: trends and developments. Lisbon: EMCDDA; 2017

[24] Kreek DM. Rationale for maintenance pharmacotherapy of opiate dependence. Research Publications-Association for Research in Nervous and Mental Disease. 1992;**70**:205-230

[25] Kreek MJ. Medical safety, side effects and toxicity of methadone. In: Proceedings of the Fourth National Conference on Methadone Treatment. . New York: National Association for the Prevention of Addiction to Narcotics. 2007. pp. 171-174

[26] Kreek MJ. Medical safety and side effects of methadone in tolerant individuals. JAMA. 1973;**223**(6):665-668

[27] Kreek MJ. Using methadone effectively: Achieving goals by application of laboratory, clinical, and evaluation research and by development of innovative programs. In: Pickens R, Leukefeld C, Schuster CR, editors. Improving Drug Abuse Treatment. National Institute on Drug Abuse Research Monograph 106. Washington, DC: Supt. of Docs., U.S. Govt. Print. Off.; 1991. pp. 245-266

[28] Gottheil E, Sterling RC, Weinstein SP. Diminished illicit drug use as a consequence of long-term methadone maintenance. Journal of Addictive Diseases. 1993;**12**(4):45-57

[29] Kleber HD. Methadone maintenance 4 decades later: Thousands of lives saved but still controversial. Journal of the American Medical Association. 2008;**300**(19):2303-2305

[30] Metzger DS, Woody GE, McLellan AT, O'brien CP, Druley P, Navaline H, et al. Human immunodeficiency virus seroconversion among intravenous drug users in-and out-of-treatment: An 18-month prospective follow-up. Journal of Acquired Immune Deficiency Syndromes. 1993;**6**:1049-1049

[31] Novick DM, Salsitz EA, Joseph H, Kreek MJ. Methadone medical maintenance: An early 21st-century perspective. Journal of Addictive Diseases. 2015;**34**(2-3):226-237

[32] Novick T, Liu Y, Alvanzo A, Zonderman AB, Evans MK, Crews DC. Lifetime cocaine and opiate use and chronic kidney disease. American Journal of Nephrology. 2016;**44**(6):447-453

[33] Kreek MJ. Methadone-related opioid agonist pharmacotherapy for heroin addiction: History, recent molecular and neurochemical research and future in mainstream medicine. Annals of the New York Academy of Sciences. 2000;**909**(1):186-216

[34] Specka M, Finkbeiner T, Lodemann E, Leifert K, Kluwig J, Gastpar M. Cognitive-motor performance of methadone-maintained patients. European Addiction Research. 2000;**6**(1):8-19

[35] Nielsen S, Larance B, Degenhardt L, Gowing L, Kehler C, Lintzeris N. Opioid agonist treatment for pharmaceutical opioid dependent people. Cochrane Database of Systematic Reviews. 2016;(5):1-65. Artical No: CD011117

[36] Cushman P, Kreek MJ, Gordis E. Ethanol and methadone in man: A possible drug interaction. Drug & Alcohol Dependence. 1978;**3**(1):35-42

[37] Kreek MJ, Garfield JW, Gutjahr CL, Giusti LM. Rifampin-induced methadone withdrawal. New England Journal of Medicine. 1976;**294**(20):1104-1106

[38] Kreek MJ. Opioid interactions with alcohol. Advances in Alcohol & Substance Abuse. 1984;**3**(4):35-46

[39] Tong TG, Pond SM, Kreek MJ, Jaffery NF, Benowitz NL. Phenytoin-induced methadone withdrawal. Annals of Internal Medicine. 1981;**94**(3):349-351

[40] Bliesener N, Albrecht S, Schwager A, Weckbecker K, Lichtermann D, Klingmuller D. Plasma testosterone and sexual function in men receiving buprenorphine maintenance for opioid dependence. The Journal of Clinical Endocrinology & Metabolism. 2005;**90**(1):203-206

[41] Hallinan R, Byrne A, Agho K, McMahon C, Tynan P, Attia J. Erectile dysfunction in men receiving methadone and buprenorphine maintenance treatment. The Journal of Sexual Medicine. 2008;**5**(3):684-692

[42] Justo D, Gal-Oz A, Paran Y, Goldin Y, Zeltser D. Methadone-associated Torsades de Pointes (polymorphic ventricular tachycardia) in opioid-dependent patients. Addiction. 2006;**101**(9):1333-1338

[43] Katchman AN, McGroary KA, Kilborn MJ, Kornick CA, Manfredi PL, Woosley RL, et al. Influence of opioid agonists on cardiac human ether-a-go-go-related gene K+ currents. Journal of Pharmacology and Experimental Therapeutics. 2002;**303**(2):688-694

[44] Ullmann R. Opiate maintenance treatment in primary health care in Germany. Heroin Addiction and Related Clinical Problems. 2010;**12**(4):53-56

[45] Johnson RE, Jaffe JH, Fudala PJ. A controlled trial of buprenorphine treatment for opioid dependence. JAMA. 1992;**267**(20):2750-2755

[46] Dahan A, Yassen A, Bijl H, Romberg R, Sarton E, Teppema L, et al. Comparison of the respiratory effects of intravenous buprenorphine and fentanyl in humans and rats. British Journal of Anaesthesia. 2005;**94**(6):825-834

[47] Mauger S, Fraser R, Gill K. Utilizing buprenorphine–naloxone to treat illicit

and prescription-opioid dependence. Neuropsychiatric Disease and Treatment. 2014;**10**:587

[48] Kraus ML, Alford DP, Kotz MM, Levounis P, Mandell TW, Meyer M, et al. Statement of the American Society of addiction medicine consensus panel on the use of buprenorphine in office-based treatment of opioid addiction. Journal of Addiction Medicine. 2011;**5**(4):254-263

[49] Correia CJ, Walsh SL, Bigelow GE, Strain EC. Effects associated with double-blind omission of buprenorphine/naloxone over a 98-h period. Psychopharmacology. 2006;**189**(3):297-306

[50] Bart G. Maintenance medication for opiate addiction: The foundation of recovery. Journal of Addictive Diseases. 2012;**31**(3):207-225

[51] Thomas CP, Fullerton CA, Kim M, Montejano L, Lyman DR, Dougherty RH, et al. Medication-assisted treatment with buprenorphine: Assessing the evidence. Psychiatric Services. 2014;**65**(2):158-170

[52] Kakko J, Svanborg KD, Kreek MJ, Heilig M. 1-year retention and social function after buprenorphine-assisted relapse prevention treatment for heroin dependence in Sweden: A randomised, placebo-controlled trial. The Lancet. 2013;**361**(9358):662-668

[53] Weiss RD, Potter JS, Fiellin DA, Byrne M, Connery HS, Dickinson W, et al. Adjunctive counseling during brief and extended buprenorphine-naloxone treatment for prescription opioid dependence: A 2-phase randomized controlled trial. Archives of General Psychiatry. 2011;**68**(12):1238-1246

[54] Amato L, Davoli M, Perucci CA, Ferri M, Faggiano F, Mattick RP. An overview of systematic reviews of the effectiveness of opiate maintenance therapies: Available evidence to inform clinical practice and research. Journal of Substance Abuse Treatment. 2005;**28**(4):321-329

[55] Mattick RP, Kimber J, Breen C, Davoli M. Buprenorphine maintenance versus placebo or methadone maintenance for opioid dependence. Cochrane Database of Systematic Reviews. 2008;**2**(2):1-48

[56] Minozzi S, Amato L, Bellisario C, Ferri M, Davoli M. Maintenance agonist treatments for opiate-dependent pregnant women. Cochrane Database of Systematic Reviews. 2013;(12). Artical No: CD006318

[57] Parran TV, Adelman CA, Merkin B, Pagano ME, Defranco R, Ionescu RA, et al. Long-term outcomes of office-based buprenorphine/naloxone maintenance therapy. Drug & Alcohol Dependence. 2010;**106**(1):56-60

[58] Schwarz R, Zelenev A, Bruce RD, Altice FL. Retention on buprenorphine treatment reduces emergency department utilization, but not hospitalization, among treatment-seeking patients with opioid dependence. Journal of Substance Abuse Treatment. 2012;**43**(4):451-457

[59] Bukten A, Skurtveit S, Gossop M, Waal H, Stangeland P, Havnes I, et al. Engagement with opioid maintenance treatment and reductions in crime: A longitudinal national cohort study. Addiction. 2012;**107**(2):393-399

[60] Douglas R, Moody DE, Chodkowski D, Andrews L, Fang WB, Morrison J, et al. Pharmacokinetic interactions between buprenorphine/naloxone and raltegravir in subjects receiving chronic buprenorphine/naloxone treatment. The American Journal of Drug and Alcohol Abuse. 2013;**39**(2):80-85

[61] Gruber VA, Rainey PM, Moody DE, Morse GD, Ma Q, Prathikanti S, et al.

Interactions between buprenorphine and the protease inhibitors darunavir-ritonavir and fosamprenavir-ritonavir. Clinical Infectious Diseases. 2011;**54**(3):414-423

[62] Soyka M. Buprenorphine use in pregnant opioid users: A critical review. CNS Drugs. 2012;**27**(8):653-662

[63] Kumar R, Saadabadi A. Buprenorphine. In StatPearls. Treasure Island (FL): StatPearls Publishing LLC. 2017

[64] Mégarbane B, Hreiche R, Pirnay S, Marie N, Baud FJ. Does high-dose buprenorphine cause respiratory depression? Toxicological Reviews. 2006;**25**(2):79-85

[65] Whelan PJ, Remski K. Buprenorphine vs methadone treatment: A review of evidence in both developed and developing worlds. Journal of Neurosciences in Rural Practice. 2012;**3**(1):45

[66] O'Connor PG, Fiellin DA. Pharmacologic treatment of heroin-dependent patients. Annals of Internal Medicine. 2000;**133**(1):4

[67] Martin WR. Naloxone. Annals of Internal Medicine. 1976;**85**:765-768

[68] Degenhardt L, Bucello C, Mathers B, Briegleb C, Ali H, Hickman M, et al. Mortality among regular or dependent users of heroin and other opioids: A systematic review and meta-analysis of cohort studies. Addiction. 2011;**106**(1):32-51

[69] Ngai SH, Berkowitz BA, Yang JC, Hempstead J, Spector S. Pharmacokinetics of naloxone in rats and in man: Basis for its potency and short duration of action. Anesthesiology, 1976;**44**(5):398-401

[70] Clark AK, Wilder CM, Winstanley EL. A systematic review of community opioid overdose prevention and naloxone distribution programs. Journal of Addiction Medicine. 2014;**8**(3):153-163

[71] McDonald R, Strang J. Are take-home naloxone programmes effective? Systematic review utilizing application of the Bradford Hill criteria. Addiction. 2016;**111**(7):1177-1187

[72] Walley AY, Xuan Z, Hackman HH, Quinn E, Doe-Simkins M, Sorensen-Alawad A, et al. Opioid overdose rates and implementation of overdose education and nasal naloxone distribution in Massachusetts: Interrupted time series analysis. BMJ. 2013;**346**:f174

[73] Horton M, McDonald R, Green TC, Nielsen S, Strang J, Degenhardt L, et al. A mapping review of take-home naloxone for people released from correctional settings. International Journal of Drug Policy. 2017;**46**:7-16

[74] Gonzalez JP, Brogden RN Naltrexone. Drugs. 1988;**35**(3): 192-213

[75] Johansson BA, Berglund M, Lindgren A. Efficacy of maintenance treatment with naltrexone for opioid dependence: A meta-analytical review. Addiction. 2006;**101**(4):491-503

[76] Kosten TR, Kreek MJ, Ragunath J, Kleber HD. A preliminary study of beta endorphin during chronic naltrexone maintenance treatment in ex-opiate addicts. Life Sciences. 1986;**39**(1):55-59

[77] Kosten TR, Kreek MJ, Ragunath J, Kleber HD. Cortisol levels during chronic naltrexone maintenance treatment in ex-opiate addicts. Biological Psychiatry. 1986;**21**(2):217-220

[78] Gonzalez G, Oliveto A, Kosten TR. Treatment of heroin (diamorphine) addiction. Drugs. 2002;**62**(9):1331-1343

[79] Gold CG, Cullen DJ, Gonzales S, Houtmeyers D, Dwyer MJ. Rapid opioid detoxification during general anesthesia a review of 20 patients. Anesthesiology: The Journal of the American Society of Anesthesiologists. 1999;**91**(6):1639-1639

[80] Bhargava HN. The effects of naltrexone on the development of physical dependence on morphine. European Journal of Pharmacology. 1978;**50**(3):193-202

[81] Kunøe N, Lobmaier P, Vederhus JK, Hjerkinn B, Hegstad S, Gossop M, et al. Retention in naltrexone implant treatment for opioid dependence. Drug & Alcohol Dependence. 2010;**111**(1):166-169

[82] Hulse GK, Morris N, Arnold-Reed D, Tait RJ. Improving clinical outcomes in treating heroin dependence: Randomized, controlled trial of oral or implant naltrexone. Archives of General Psychiatry. 2009;**66**(10):1108-1115

[83] Krupitsky E, Nunes EV, Ling W, Illeperuma A, Gastfriend DR, Silverman BL. Injectable extended-release naltrexone for opioid dependence: A double-blind, placebo-controlled, multicentre randomised trial. Lancet. 2011;**377**:1506-1513

[84] Ndegwa S, Pant S, Pohar S, Mierzwinski-Urban M. Injectable extended-release naltrexone to treat opioid use disorder. In: CADTH Issues in Emerging Health Technologies. Ottawa (ON): Canadian Agency for Drugs and Technologies in Health. 2017;163

[85] Lee JD, Nunes EV Jr, Novo P, Bachrach K, Bailey GL, Bhatt S, et al. Comparative effectiveness of extended-release naltrexone versus buprenorphine-naloxone for opioid relapse prevention (X: BOT): A multicentre, open-label, randomised controlled trial. The Lancet. 2018;**391**(10118):309-318

[86] Mattick RP, Breen C, Kimber J, Davoli M. Methadone maintenance therapy versus no opioid replacement therapy for opioid dependence. Cochrane Database of Systematic Reviews. 2009;**3**:CD002209

[87] Lee JD, Friedmann PD, Kinlock TW, et al. Extended-release naltrexone to prevent opioid relapse in criminal justice offenders. The New England Journal of Medicine. 2016;**374**:1232-1242

[88] Itzoe M, Guarnieri M. New developments in managing opioid addiction: Impact of a subdermal buprenorphine implant. Drug Design, Development and Therapy. 2017;**11**:1429

[89] Smith L, Mosley J, Johnson J, Nasri M. Probuphine (buprenorphine) subdermal implants for the treatment of opioid-dependent patients. Pharmacy and Therapeutics. 2017;**42**(8):505-508

[90] Eder H, Jagsch R, Kraigher D, Primorac A, Ebner N, Fischer G. Comparative study of the effectiveness of slow-release morphine and methadone for opioid maintenance therapy. Addiction. 2005;**100**(8):1101-1109

[91] Kraigher D, Jagsch R, Gombas W, Ortner R, Eder H, Primorac A, et al. Use of slow-release oral morphine for the treatment of opioid dependence. European Addiction Research. 2008;**11**(3):145-151

[92] Kastelic A, Dubajic G, Strbad E. Slow-release oral morphine for maintenance treatment of opioid addicts intolerant to methadone or with inadequate withdrawal suppression. Addiction. 2008;**103**(11):1837-1846

[93] Walton G, Nolan S, Sutherland C, Ahamad K. Sustained release oral morphine as an alternative to methadone for the treatment of opioid-use disorder post Torsades de Pointes

cardiac arrest. BMJ case reports. 2015. bcr2015210239

[94] Hammig R, Kohler W, Bonorden-Kleij K, et al. Safety and tolerability of slow-release oral morphine versus methadone in the treatment of opioid dependence. Journal of Substance Abuse Treatment. 2014;**47**:275-281

[95] Beck T, Haasen C, Verthein U, Walcher S, Schuler C, Backmund M, et al. Maintenance treatment for opioid dependence with slow-release oral morphine: A randomized cross-over, non-inferiority study versus methadone. Addiction. 2014;**109**(4):617-626

[96] Ferri M, Minozzi S, Bo A, Amato L. Slow-release oral morphine as maintenance therapy for opioid dependence. Cochrane Database of Systematic Reviews. 2013;(6): pp 1-30. Artical No: CD009879

[97] Gillen C, Hurand M, Kobelt DJ, Wnendt S. Affinity, potency and efficacy of tramadol and its metabolites at the cloned human μ-opioid receptor. Naunyn-Schmiedeberg's Archives of Pharmacology. 2000;**362**(2):116-121

[98] Lofwall MR, Babalonis S, Nuzzo PA, Siegel A, Campbell C, Walsh L. Efficacy of extended-release tramadol for treatment of prescription opioid withdrawal: A two-phase randomized controlled trial. Drug and Alcohol Dependence. 2013;**133**(1):188-197

[99] Dunn KE, Tompkins DA, Bigelow GE, Strain EC. Efficacy of tramadol extended-release for opioid withdrawal: A randomized clinical trial. JAMA Psychiatry. 2017;**74**(9):885-893

[100] Sarkar S, Lal R, Varshney M, Balhara YPS. Tramadol for maintenance in opioid dependence: A retrospective chart review. Journal of Opioid Management. 2017;**13**(5):329-334

[101] Heidbreder C. Rationale in support of the use of selective dopamine D3 receptor antagonists for the pharmacotherapeutic management of substance use disorders. Naunyn-Schmiedebergs Archives of Pharmacology. 2013;**386**:167-176

[102] Lai M, Chen W, Zhu H, Zhou X, Liu H, Zhang F, et al. Low dose risperidone attenuates cue-induced but not heroin-induced reinstatement of heroin seeking in an animal model of relapse. International Journal of Neuropsychopharmcology. 2013;**16**:1569-1575

[103] Almeida-Santos AF, Gobira PH, Souza DP, Ferreira RC, Romero TR, Duarte ID, et al. The antipsychotic aripiprazole selectively prevents the stimulant and rewarding effects of morphine in mice. European Journal of Pharmacology. 2014;**742**:139-144

[104] Moran LM, Phillips KA, Kowalczyk WJ, Ghitza UE, Agage DA, Epstein DH, et al. Aripiprazole for cocaine abstinence: A randomized-controlled trial with ecological momentary assessment. Behavioural Pharmacology. 2017;**28**(1):63-73

[105] Portugal GS, Al-Hasani R, Fakira AK, Gonzalez-Romero JL, Melyan Z, McCall JG, et al. Hippocampal long-term potentiation is disrupted during expression and extinction but is restored after reinstatement of morphine place preference. The Journal of Neuroscience. 2014;**34**(2):527-538

[106] Ma YY, Yu P, Guo CY, Cui CL. Effects of ifenprodil on morphine-induced conditioned place preference and spatial learning and memory in rats. Neurochemical Research. 2011;**36**(3):383-391

[107] Harris AC, Rothwell PE, Gewirtz JC. Effects of the NMDA receptor antagonist memantine on the expression and development of

acute opiate dependence as assessed by withdrawal-potentiated startle and hyperalgesia. Psychopharmacology. 2008;**196**(4):649-660

[108] Popik P, Skolnick P. The NMDA antagonist memantine blocks the expression and maintenance of morphine dependence. Pharmacology Biochemistry and Behavior. 1996;**53**(4):791-797

[109] Bisaga A, Comer SD, Ward AS, Popik P, Kleber HD, Fischman MW. The NMDA antagonist memantine attenuates the expression of opioid physical dependence in humans. Psychopharmacology. 2001;**157**(1):1-10

[110] Bisaga A, Sullivan MA, Cheng WY, Carpenter KM, Mariani JJ, Levin FR, et al. A placebo controlled trial of memantine as an adjunct to oral naltrexone for opioid dependence. Drug and Alcohol Dependence. 2011;**119**(1-2):e23-e29

[111] Bisaga A, Sullivan MA, Glass A, Mishlen K, Carpenter KM, Mariani JJ, et al. A placebo-controlled trial of memantine as an adjunct to injectable extended release naltrexone for opioid dependence. Journal of Substance Abuse Treatment. 2014;**46**:546-552

[112] Cuellar B, Fernández AP, Lizasoain I, Moro MA, Lorenzo P, Bentura ML, et al. Up-regulation of neuronal NO synthase immunoreactivity in opiate dependence and withdrawal. Psychopharmacology. 2000;**148**:66-73

[113] Kolesnikov YA, Pick CG, Ciszewska G, Pasternak GW. Blockade of tolerance to morphine but not to kappa opioids by a nitric oxide synthase inhibitor. Proceedings of the National Academy of Sciences of the United States of America. 1993;**90**:5162-5166

[114] Leza JC, Lizasoain I, Cuellar B, Moro MA, Lorenzo P. Correlation between brain nitric oxide synthase activity and opiate withdrawal. Naunyn-Schmiedeberg's Archives of Pharmacology. 1996;**353**:349-354

[115] Cousins MS, Roberts DC, de Wit H. GABAB receptor agonists for the treatment of drug addiction: A review of recent findings. Drug and Alcohol Dependence. 2002;**65**(3):209-220

[116] Brebner K, Phelan R, Roberts DC. Effect of baclofen on cocaine self-administration in rats reinforced under fixed-ratio 1 and progressive-ratio schedules. Psychopharmacology. 2000;**148**:314-321

[117] Colombo G, Agabio R, Carai MA, Lobina C, Pani M, Reali R, et al. Ability of baclofen in reducing alcohol intake and withdrawal severity: I. Preclinical evidence. Alcoholism: Clinical and Experimental Research. 2000;**24**:58-66

[118] Fattore L, Cossu G, Martellotta MC, Fratta W. Baclofen antagonizes intravenous self-administration of nicotine in mice and rats. Alcohol and Alcoholism. 2002;**37**:495-498

[119] Ranaldi R, Poeggel K. Baclofen decreases methamphetamine self-administration in rats. Neuroreport. 2002;**13**:1107-1110

[120] Bexis S, Ong J, White J. Attenuation of morphine withdrawal signs by the GABA(B) receptor agonist baclofen. Life Sciences. 2001;**70**:395-401

[121] Zarrindast MR, Mousa-Ahmadi E. Effects of GABAergic system on naloxone-induced jumping in morphine-dependent mice. European Journal of Pharmacology. 1999;**381**:129-133

[122] Meng S, Quan W, Qi X, Su Z, Yang S. Effect of baclofen on morphine-induced conditioned place preference, extinction, and stress-induced reinstatement in chronically

stressed mice. Psychopharmacology. 2014;**231**:27-36

[123] Assadi SM, Radgoodarzi R, Ahmadi-Abhari SA. Baclofen for maintenance treatment of opioid dependence: A randomized double-blind placebo-controlled clinical trial [ISRCTN32121581]. BMC Psychiatry. 2003;**3**(1):16

[124] Pitkänen A, Kharatishvili I, Narkilahti S, Lukasiuk K, Nissinen J. Administration of diazepam during status epilepticus reduces development and severity of epilepsy in rat. Epilepsy Research. 2005;**63**:27-42

[125] Cheng JK, Lee SZ, Yang JR, Wang CH, Liao YY, Chen CC, et al. Does gabapentin act as an agonist at native GABA B receptors? Journal of Biomedical Science. 2004;**11**(3):346-355

[126] Cunningham MO, Woodhall GL, Thompson SE, Dooley DJ, Jones RS. Dual effects of gabapentin and pregabalin on glutamate release at rat entorhinal synapses in vitro. European Journal of Neuroscience. 2004;**20**(6):1566-1576

[127] Hasanein P, Shakeri S. Pregabalin role in inhibition of morphine analgesic tolerance and physical dependency in rats. European Journal of Pharmacology. 2014;**742**:113-117

[128] Bao YH, Zhou QH, Chen R, Xu H, Zeng L, Zhang X, et al. Gabapentin attenuates morphine tolerance through interleukin-10. Neuroreport. 2014;**25**(2):71-76

[129] Sanders NC, Mancino MJ, Gentry WB, Guise JB, Bickel WK, Thostenson J, et al. Randomized, placebo-controlled pilot trial of gabapentin during an outpatient, buprenorphine-assisted detoxification procedure. Experimental and Clinical Psychopharmacology. 2013;**21**(4):294-302

[130] Muldoon PP, Jackson KJ, Perez E, Harenza JL, Molas S, Rais B, et al. The $\alpha 3\beta 4^*$ nicotinic ACh receptor subtype mediates physical dependence to morphine: Mouse and human studies. British Journal of Pharmacology. 2014;**171**(16):3845-3857

[131] Hooten WM, Warner DO. Varenicline for opioid withdrawal in patients with chronic pain: A randomized, single-blinded, placebo controlled pilot trial. Addictive Behaviors. 2015;**42**:69-72

[132] Sharifipour M, Izadpanah E, Nikkhoo B, Zare S, Abdolmaleki A, Hassanzadeh K, et al. A new pharmacological role for donepezil: Attenuation of morphine-induced tolerance and apoptosis in rat central nervous system. Journal of Biomedical Science. 2014;**21**(1):6

[133] Gawel K, Labuz K, Jenda M, Silberring J, Kotlinska JH. Influence of cholinesterase inhibitors, donepezil and rivastigmine on the acquisition, expression, and reinstatement of morphine-induced conditioned place preference in rats. Behavioural Brain Research. 2014;**268**:169-176

[134] Scavone JL, Sterling RC, Van Bockstaele EJ. Cannabinoid and opioid interactions: Implications for opiate dependence and withdrawal. Neuroscience. 2013;**248**:637-654

[135] Hurd YL, Yoon M, Manini AF, Hernandez S, Olmedo R, Ostman M, et al. Early phase in the development of cannabidiol as a treatment for addiction: Opioid relapse takes initial center stage. Neurotherapeutics. 2015;**12**(4):807-815

[136] Mechoulam R, Peters M, Murillo-Rodriguez E, Hanus LO. Cannabidiol—Recent advances. Chemistry & Biodiversity. 2007;**4**:1678-1692

[137] Thomas A, Baillie GL, Phillips AM, et al. Cannabidiol displays unexpectedly

high potency as an antagonist of CB1 and CB2 receptor agonists in vitro. British Journal of Pharmacology. 2007;**150**:613-623

[138] Ren Y, Whittard J, Higuera-Matas A, Morris CV, Hurd YL. Cannabidiol, a nonpsychotropic component of cannabis, inhibits cue-induced heroin seeking and normalizes discrete mesolimbic neuronal disturbances. Journal of Neuroscience. 2009;**29**(47):14764-14769

[139] Katsidoni V, Anagnostou I, Panagis G. Cannabidiol inhibits the reward-facilitating effect of morphine: Involvement of 5-HT1A receptors in the dorsal raphe nucleus. Addiction Biology. 2013;**18**:286-296

[140] Manini AF, Yiannoulos G, Bergamaschi MM, Hernandez S, Olmedo R, Barnes AJ, et al. Safety and pharmacokinetics of oral cannabidiol when administered concomitantly with intravenous fentanyl in humans. Journal of Addiction Medicine. 2015;**9**(3):204

[141] Harricharan R, Abboussi O, Daniels WM. Addiction: A dysregulation of satiety and inflammatory processes. Progress in Brain Research. 2017;**235**:65-91

[142] Coller JK, Hutchinson MR. Implications of central immune signaling caused by drugs of abuse: Mechanisms, mediators and new therapeutic approaches for prediction and treatment of drug dependence. Pharmacology & Therapeutics. 2012;**134**(2):219-245

[143] Cunha-Oliveira T, Rego AC, Garrido J, Borges F, Macedo T, Oliveira CR. Neurotoxicity of heroin–cocaine combinations in rat cortical neurons. Toxicology. 2010;**276**(1):11-17

[144] Fecho K, Maslonek KA, Dykstra LA, Lysle DT. Assessment of the involvement of central nervous system and peripheral opioid receptors in the immunomodulatory effects of acute morphine treatment in rats. The Journal of Pharmacology and Experimental Therapeutics. 1996;**276**(2):626-636

[145] McCarthy L, Wetzel M, Sliker JK, Eisenstein TK, Rogers TJ. Opioids, opioid receptors, and the immune response. Drug and Alcohol Dependence. 2001;**62**(2):111-123

[146] Raghavendra V, Tanga F, DeLeo JA. Inhibition of microglial activation attenuates the development but not existing hypersensitivity in a rat model of neuropathy. The Journal of Pharmacology and Experimental Therapeutics. 2003;**306**(2):624-630

[147] Chen SL, Tao PL, Chu CH, Chen SH, Wu HE, Tseng LF, et al. Low-dose memantine attenuated morphine addictive behavior through its anti-inflammation and neurotrophic effects in rats. Journal of Neuroimmune Pharmacology. 2012;**37**(4):393-398

[148] Eisch AJ, Barrot M, Schad CA, Self DW, Nestler EJ. Opiates inhibit neurogenesis in the adult rat hippocampus. Proceedings of the National Academy of Sciences of the United States of America. 2000;**97**(13):7579-7584

[149] Campbell LA, Avdoshina V, Rozzi S, Mocchetti I. CCL5 and cytokine expression in the rat brain: Differential modulation by chronic morphine and morphine withdrawal. Brain, Behaviour and Immunity. 2013;**34**:130-140

[150] Theberge FR, Li X, Kambhampati S, Pickens CL, Laurent RS, Bossert JM, et al. Effect of chronic delivery of the toll-like receptor 4 antagonist (+)-naltrexone on incubation of heroin craving. Biological Psychiatry. 2013;**73**(8):729-737

[151] Mattioli TA, Leduc-Pessah H, Skelhorne-Gross G, Nicol CJ, Milne B, Trang T, et al. Toll-like receptor 4 mutant and null mice retain morphine-induced tolerance, hyperalgesia, and physical dependence. PLoS One. 2014;**9**(5):e97361

[152] Yamagata T, Ichinose M. Agents against cytokine synthesis or receptors. European Journal of Pharmacology. 2006;**533**(1):289-301

[153] Mizuno T, Kurotani T, Komatsu Y, Kawanokuchi J, Kato H, Mitsuma N, et al. Neuroprotective role of phosphodiesterase inhibitor ibudilast on neuronal cell death induced by activated microglia. Neuropharmacology. 2004;**6**(3):404-411

[154] Cooper ZD, Johnson KW, Pavlicova M, Glass A, Vosburg SK, Sullivan MA, et al. The effects of ibudilast, a glial activation inhibitor, on opioid withdrawal symptoms in opioid dependent volunteers. Addiction Biology. 2016;**21**(4):895-903

[155] Ray LA, Roche DJ, Heinzerling K, Shoptaw S. Opportunities for the development of neuroimmune therapies in addiction. International Review of Neurobiology. 2014;**118**:381-401

[156] de Guglielmo G, Melis M, De Luca MA, Kallupi M, Li HW, Niswender K, et al. PPAR gamma activation attenuates opioid consumption and modulates mesolimbic dopamine transmission. Neuropsychopharmacology. 2015;**40**:927-937

[157] Melis M, Carta S, Fattore L, Tolu S, Yasar S, Goldberg SR, et al. Peroxisome proliferator-activated receptors-alpha modulate dopamine cell activity through nicotinic receptors. Biological Psychiatry. 2010;**68**(3):256-264

[158] Ghavimi H, Azarfardian A, Maleki-Dizaji N, Hassanzadeh K, Ghanbarzadeh S, Charkhpour M. Acute administration of pioglitazone attenuates morphine withdrawal syndrome in rat: A novel role of pioglitazone. Drug Research. 2015;**65**:113-118

[159] Crist RC, Clarke TK, Ang A, Ambrose-Lanci LM, Lohoff FW, Saxon AJ, et al. An intronic variant in OPRD1 predicts treatment outcome for opioid dependence in African-Americans. Neuropsychopharmacology. 2013;**38**:2003-2010

[160] Barratt DT, Coller JK, Hallinan R, Byrne A, White JM, Foster DJ, et al. ABCB1 haplotype and OPRM1 118A>G genotype interaction in methadone maintenance treatment pharmacogenetics. Pharmacogenomics and Personalized Medicine. 2012;**5**:53-62

[161] Gerra G, Somaini L, Leonardi C, Cortese E, Maremmani I, Manfredini M, et al. Association between gene variants and response to buprenorphine maintenance treatment. Psychiatry Research. 2014;**215**:202-207

[162] Brockmöller J, Tzvetkov MV. Pharmacogenetics: Data, concepts and tools to improve drug discovery and drug treatment. European Journal of Clinical Pharmacology. 2008;**64**(2):133-157

[163] Dolinoy DC. Epigenetic gene regulation: Early environmental exposures. Pharmacogenomics. 2007;**8**:5-10

[164] Kronfol MM, Dozmorov MG, Huang R, Slattum PW, McClay JL. The role of epigenomics in personalized medicine. Expert Review of Precision Medicine and Drug Development. 2017;**2**(1):33-45

[165] Nielsen DA, Utrankar A, Reyes JA, Simons DD, Kosten TR. Epigenetics of drug abuse: Predisposition or response. Pharmacogenomics. 2012;**13**:1149-1160

[166] Nielsen DA, Hamon S, Yuferov V, Jackson C, Ho A, Ott J, et al. Ethnic diversity of DNA methylation in the OPRM1 promoter region in lymphocytes of heroin addicts. Human Genetics. 2010;**127**:639-649

[167] Chorbov VM, Todorov AA, Lynskey MT, Cicero TJ. Elevated levels of DNA methylation at the OPRM1 promoter in blood and sperm from male opioid addicts. Journal of Opioid Management. 2011;7:258-264

[168] Modesto-Lowe V, Swiezbin K, Chaplin M, Hoefer G. Use and misuse of opioid agonists in opioid addiction. Cleveland Clinic Journal of Medicine. 2017;**84**(5):377-384